T0187450

EMPOWERMENT
IN HEALTH
AND WELLNESS

EDITED BY
ANDREW A PARSONS, SUE JACKSON,
JACKIE ARNOLD

Empowerment in Health and Wellness

First published in 2021 by

Panoma Press Ltd
48 St Vincent Drive, St Albans, Herts, AL1 5SJ, UK
info@panomapress.com
www.panomapress.com

Book layout by Neil Coe.

978-1-784529-29-1

The rights of Gavin Andrews, Jackie Arnold, Victoria Hamilton, Enrico Illuminati, Sue Jackson, Aga Kehinde, Ann Lewis, Silvia Mirandola, Andrew A Parsons, Fiona Stimson, Chris Ullman and Amanda White to be identified as the authors of this work have been asserted in accordance with sections 77 and 78 of the Copyright, Designs and Patents Act 1988.

A CIP catalogue record for this book is available from the British Library.

TESTIMONIALS

"The coaching service has taken the Fountain Centre to a new level of support for patients, families and carers living with and beyond cancer. This book shares the professionalism, deep expertise and collaborative nature of this innovative volunteer service."

Anne Pike, State Registered Occupational Therapist, Head of the Fountain Centre and the Surrey and Sussex Co Clinical Lead for personalised care and support (cancer)

"Empowerment in Health and Wellness offers a rich and engaging read, drawn from a breadth of complementary and differing professional perspectives. Being informed by both experience and expertise, it is practical in nature: through accessible language, clearly introduced concepts and illustrative examples. Moreover, it is comprehensive in form, exploring a broad range of topics that extends our appreciation in this arena. Each chapter provides gifts of insight for us to weave into our understanding and draw upon to inform our practice. I would recommend this book as being a go-to reference guide within the field of health and wellbeing."

Dr Cathy Brown, Chartered Occupational Psychologist, Organisational Development Consultant and Writer

"This is a much needed, holistic mind-body-spirit approach to health that provides practical guidance to enable us to take highly motivated purpose-led actions that are sustainable. A must-read for all healthcare practitioners that want to take their impact to the next level, this book shows us how to better manage our wellbeing, develop deeper relationships with ourselves and with others and ultimately lead more fulfilling lives through taking control in whatever situation we find ourselves."

**Dr Monika Misra, Occupational Medicine Physician, UK
MBBS, MRCGP, MFOM, MSc Nutritional Medicine**

"We live in uncertain times. Life no longer functions as it did before and we are thrown back on ourselves. At the same time this time brings many possibilities. It is a question of how to look at it – as an opportunity or a problem. This book offers a wonderful overview of how to ground yourself, to empower and motivate yourself to move forward. It shows tips and tricks both for private and professional use on what it takes to thrive in this challenging time. It has something for everyone and considers the uniqueness of everyone. I can highly recommend it."

**Dr Christa Uehlinger, Intercultural Coach,
Owner, Christa Uehlinger Linking People**

"Having worked as a nurse for a long time in cancer care and now as a coach I was interested to read how the authors of Empowerment in Health and Wellness used coaching principles and approaches in their work with people with cancer. The book was easy to read with chapters that you could dip in and out of depending on your interest. The holistic approach and the information from the perspectives of different professionals in this area made it much more than just a coaching book, which would be of interest to people with cancer as well as the people that treat and care for them. I like the practical and easy to apply Top Tips at the end of each chapter which makes the book a very useful addition to anyone with an interest in how to put coaching into practice in daily life for an improvement in health and wellbeing."

Amy Sinacola, RGN, ICF ACC Wellbeing Coach

ACKNOWLEDGEMENTS

We gratefully acknowledge the support of the Luigi Francescon Trust in the publication of this manuscript.

We also thank the staff and supporters of the Fountain Centre including all the coaches (past and present) who have given time and support in building the service.

PREFACE

About the book

The aim of this book is to share a distillation of professional and practical coaching skills, experiences, resources and our learning in supporting people to develop and thrive during challenging situations. We have witnessed the positive impact coaching and mentoring makes in such diverse transitions as dealing with a life-changing medical situation to adapting to new roles and challenges in the workplace. The authors have a variety of training and backgrounds and all have an interest in enabling the optimal health and wellness of individuals. The majority of authors are part of the volunteer team providing coaching for cancer patients and their families at the Fountain Centre, St Luke's Cancer Centre, Royal Surrey Foundation Trust, UK. Some of the coaches provide support to other charities and social enterprises.

Our coaching team are all members of at least one professional body and our work aligns with the definitions of coaching and the Ethical Frameworks from the International Coaching Federation, the Association for Coaching and the European Mentoring Coaching Council.

Experienced health professionals have contributed to provide allied, additional and valued input to enhance the information available to support comprehensive health and wellness.

Our objectives for the book are to share information, practical case studies and sustainable skills and resources for professionals involved in the support of health both in healthcare settings and workplaces.

The limitations of this book

This book is not intended as an evidence-based intervention guide. Much of the work conducted by the coaches has been led by our own evidence-based practice, and specific randomised controlled clinical trials have not been conducted.

This book is not concerned with specific interventions to induce behavioural changes in individuals or build modalities of resilience. Rather its aim is to share our experiences, approaches, reflections and feedback to support and enhance self-regulation for that most important of human attributes, health.

Our professional practice extends across different cultures and organisations. However, the academic and evidence-based practice understanding of coaching and mentoring across cultures is a developing expertise. These areas are also not specifically covered in this book.

This book includes a selection of important topics to enhance health and wellness. Additional topics, for example physical fitness and social relationships, are not covered specifically and resources for these may be found elsewhere.

The Fountain Centre Coaching Service

The Fountain Cancer Care Centre was established in 1998 and in 2001 became a registered charity. The Fountain Centre (est. 1998) (www.fountaincentre.org) is an independent charity that supports anyone impacted by cancer under the medical care of St Luke's Cancer Centre covering 1.3 million people across Surrey, Sussex and Hampshire. The charity is located within the grounds of the hospital and provides supportive services such as access to information, delivering complementary therapies and providing emotional support through counselling and coaching. In addition, there is also a family service supporting children of patients.

The coaching service was established in 2014 with the support of Eugenia Olavide, a Reiki practitioner and certified professional medical coach. Eugenia and the Fountain Centre identified a gap for cancer patients to develop skills to manage the challenges of living with and beyond cancer that were not being met by other psychological interventions. Soon after, Eugenia was joined by Andrew Parsons, a fellow medical coach, and supported by the Fountain Centre team developed the service around different coaching modalities and established a clear and robust governance structure. The coaching service is an example of social innovation with eight professionally trained volunteer coaches who as a collective were inspired to contribute to this book.

CONTENTS

PART 2   Information   73

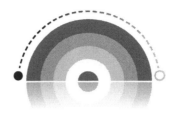

CHAPTER 1

CHANGE AND COMPLEXITY: CHALLENGES TO HEALTH AND WELLNESS

Sue Jackson, Jackie Arnold and Andrew A Parsons

Personal and professional life and health today is very different from the last century. Medical science has given us significant disease control, increased life expectancy and health benefits. However, at the same time modern lifestyles and the environment contribute to new health challenges.

Health is much more than the absence of disease. The World Health Organization's definition of health creates an aspirational state of complete mental, physical and social wellbeing. As a consequence, developing a framework for health requires a focus on individual, environmental and societal issues, as these all impact our sense of wellbeing. The determinants of individual health include physical (eg bodily fitness), mental (eg sense of coherence) and social (eg access to services, supportive relationships) dimensions. The environmental and societal determinants include diverse social structures (eg community and family – genetic factors and early years), ecological considerations (eg pollution and climate change) and economic factors (eg financial, income).

The National Wellness Institute defines wellness as 'an active process through which people become aware of, and make choices towards, a more successful existence. Wellness is holistic and multidimensional and includes emotional, occupational, physical, spiritual, intellectual and social aspects.'

The impact of the COVID-19 pandemic in our global, technologically connected lives will take time to establish.

In managing the aftermath of the pandemic and with the possibilities of its recurrence, society faces a whole range of complex issues and environmental, technological, social and personal challenges. As changes take place it seems certain our world is much more volatile, uncertain, complex and ambiguous (VUCA) within all the different contexts of our lives. The economic upheaval and uncertainty will require us to adapt rapidly and with skill to maintain our health and wellness. These conditions, which occur in the context of continual change, and involve multiple stakeholders each with different priorities, are known as Wicked Problems. These need different ways of thinking and action to resolve them.

Our experience of coaching with people living with and beyond cancer has provided transferable skills which we use to support people in mental health and professional contexts.

In this book we refer to the people we support differently depending on the practitioner's context. In coaching, we use the term 'individuals' for the people we support; in the medical profession they are 'patients'. We have kept the differences to respect these contexts. Where the term 'individual' appears, it can, as appropriate, be substituted by clinicians and healthcare practitioners for 'patient' and by coaches for 'client' or 'coachee'.

Empowerment defined

Empowerment is an important concept for healthcare as it results in people being more able to self-manage their situation and exert greater influence on their determinants of health.

"To empower is to enable."

There are different perspectives on empowerment and Freire's definition below provides some insight into the elements of empowerment from an educational perspective.

"The practice of freedom, the means by which men and women deal critically with reality and discover how to participate in the transformation of their world." (Paolo Freire, 1993)

Freire wrote extensively about educational paradigms that enable people. He suggests there are no neutral educational programmes; they either strive to create conformity to an ideal or they enable the practice of freedom. Freire believed empowering elements enabling freedom can be developed in an educational setting by critical dialogue and collaboration. As the coaching process facilitates participation, learning and development there is an opportunity for practitioners to support the development of empowerment.

A diagrammatic representation of this cycle of empowerment provides a learning process model for coaches, in collaborative dialogue with their individuals or patients, to enquire, explore, implement actions and review.

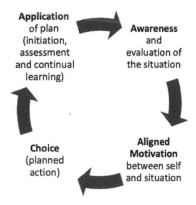

Figure 1: The Cycle of Empowerment

Heightening critical awareness supports people to notice, broaden perspectives and make an active assessment of where they are currently and exploring where they want or might want to go next. In our experience as coaches, this requires an alignment of internal and external motivations in an active sharing or collaboration with others to move towards choice. These motivations drive the development of planned actions and strategies which can then be implemented. Critical awareness and review of the results of this implementation completes and restarts the process.

This cycle therefore provides a way for the coach to support their individual (or patient) to learn and adapt to their new environment or situation. The focus for the coaching dialogue can explore both the individual and environmental determinants of health and, depending on the knowledge and skills of the coach, provide the individual with deep insights, different perspectives and a sense of enablement.

Coaching enables learning and empowerment

In *Beyond Goals* (2013), Spence & Deci define excellence in coaching as:

"The implementation of a set of interpersonal processes that lead to the coachee experiencing enhanced physical health (physiological), engagement in effective, purposeful actions (behavioural), the possession of sufficient attentional control to process information effectively (cognitive), an ability to encounter a wider range of

emotional states with equanimity and poise (affective), and the conscious linking of personal goals and commitments to important beliefs, core values, and/or developing interests (meaning)."

Therefore, coaches and professionals use coaching skills to support individuals to satisfy the basic psychological needs for the benefit of their physical, mental, emotional and spiritual health. Individuals learn how to develop their potential to improve their health in whatever circumstances they find themselves.

Coaching engages individuals in a process that builds and generates feelings of:

- Competence to act on and expand their capabilities

- Relatedness in the ways they connect with others

- Autonomy; promoting their ability to self-regulate and develop mindsets, motivations and behaviours that are more integrated psychologically

These increase the individual's level of self-determination.

An increase in self-determination in coaching promotes the individual's sense of empowerment. This is one potential outcome of coaching. In our experience, the need to feel more empowered in different aspects of their lives is a common theme for people facing life-changing health or professional situations. The sense of moving beyond a diagnosis, reconfiguring life after treatment and/or developing a sense of confidence and capability in challenging roles often derives from the individual becoming empowered in the situation. Coaching for Empowerment in Health and Wellness is almost always much more than reaching goals. The Spence & Deci definition of coaching (above) is a cornerstone to developing the scope of coaching for empowerment. Coaching is a collaborative dialogue that encompasses a range of approaches which enhance critical awareness of behaviours, feelings, intentions and attitudes (beliefs and values). It generates motivation to expand choice, precipitate action and promote ongoing learning and emotional agility.

Through our coaching experience and co-supervision, the Fountain Centre coaches have identified three core coaching pillars involved in supporting health and wellness empowerment:

1. Engaging greater **awareness** (of and for self/others)

2. Providing **information** (eg feedback or psycho-educational or self-help tools)

3. Creating a **learning** environment

We have discovered that these pillars provide the foundations for individuals in challenging health situations to make proactive choices to promote their health and make progress in determining what is important in their lives and move towards their new beginnings, living with and beyond their diagnoses.

This book is structured to reflect these three pillars of coaching for health and wellness empowerment. The framework of empowerment creates the safe, confidential and trusting alliance for individuals to develop their new ways of being, appropriate for their changing health or professional situation.

Part 1: **Awareness**: ways we can improve our health by noticing, connecting with ourselves and acting with intention.

This section includes personal and professional case studies reflecting on resources to manage our thoughts, feelings and emotions and stay present and grounded. This engagement increases our sense of connection, which helps to support the flow of our energy. We become more focused on our thoughts and in our bodies, paying attention to what emerges from coaching conversations, energetic practices, contact with nature and our spiritual dimension. This section includes the importance of raising awareness to take pre-emptive measures to boost our immune systems, maintain balance and imbed strategies for optimal health.

Part 2: **Information**: the processes we can use to support the health of others.

This section begins with a personal leadership approach to health through a framework for coaching conversations on the narratives of being healthy. An outline of the 3-Talk method for healthcare practitioners follows and illustrates ways to create shared decision making to build on and improve patients' outcomes.

This is complemented by a chapter on the importance of the attitudes needed to create a learning environment with individuals from a clinical perspective. Measures of optimal health are then discussed as a way for us to gain information on our current health status and monitor our progress. The valuable biofeedback approaches to maintain physiological and emotional coherence are also discussed.

Part 3: **Learning**: the importance of the implementation of insights developed from expanding awareness or seeking information.

Gathering feedback, developing new skills and the role of reflection in learning for practitioners are essential elements of coaching supervision. In this section we explore an approach to ensure we manage the boundaries and ethical issues of our practice, experience and development.

Our final chapter brings together the three pillars with thoughts, reflections and questions to create sustainable learning and development. This is important whether you are a coach practitioner concerned with health empowerment in the coaching process, or an individual interested in ways to enhance your health.

Each chapter includes information, experiences and Top Tips for you to employ either with individuals or personally to nurture your complete health – physical, mental, emotional and spiritual. It is important, in our experience, that coaches and healthcare practitioners engage with awareness in (or attend to) their self-care for their personal benefit and to serve the professional relationship.

In presenting our knowledge and experience with you we have three objectives:

1. To share skills and learning to enhance the work and impact of healthcare professionals in the service of their individuals.

2. To help improve community health and wellbeing in alignment with the UN Global Goals (Goal 3: Good Health and Wellbeing).

3. That our coming together as a group of professionals in the production of this book heightens our own skills and has positive impacts at the Fountain Centre for those individuals living with and beyond cancer and their families.

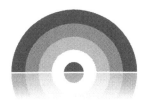

PART 1:
AWARENESS

In this section, the reader is taken on a journey of exploration and learning. You will discover some of the well-researched resources available to practitioners for supporting themselves and their individuals. The essence of each chapter is to bring a heightened level of non-judgmental attention and presence to what is happening in the body, mind and soul.

Compassionate enquiry into and learning from experience increases resourcefulness, autonomy and empowerment. This benefits an individual's health, wellness, motivation and capacity to master self-management.

As practitioners it is important for us to realise that we are on the parallel journey of our clients in developing our own empowerment in health and wellness.

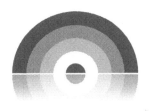

CHAPTER 2

PRESENCE AND MINDFULNESS

Jackie Arnold

When working at our best there is a heart connection created at a fundamentally deep level. This enables us to work on the true nature of the issues that arise and support others to achieve insights by means of safe exploration.

This chapter explores the way in which you are able to create a safe space and mindful presence, for self and others, to nurture a genuine quality of present moment attention. This chapter will also cover the importance of our voice tone, flexibility and pace in addition to the essential alignment of our body (mind-heart-gut).

As coaching professionals, we attempt to show ways to be present in the here and now coming from a place of acceptance and non-judgment. By increasing levels of attention, it becomes possible to co-create a deep thinking and being space for the individual to reflect and grow.

"The inner self is revealed in the unconscious language and symbolic landscape we create." Jackie Arnold, *Coaching Skills for Leaders in the Workplace (2017)*

Research proves that mindfulness practice boosts happiness and wellbeing and can also increase levels of attention and empathy.

Everything has an energy, even inanimate objects. You create an energy flow between you and anyone you come into contact with, and you can also affect their energy in either an empowering or negative way. Ideally you understand how important it is to sense and tap into another person's energy field while at the same time being aware of your own patterns of thought, cultural influence and energy flow. Ensuring your head, heart and gut are aligned, balanced, grounded and positive helps to create a similar energy in your individuals. This is an essential step into health empowerment allowing others their own space and world view.

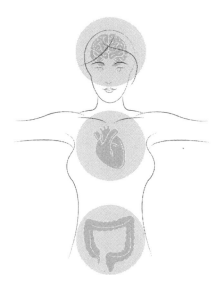

Figure 2: The balance of head, heart and gut

Mindfulness-inspired exercise

One of the ways in which this balance can be achieved for both practitioner and individual is to practise slow breathing to gain guidance from the gut and heart areas.

Sitting comfortably in a peaceful environment, begin to breathe slowly from the gut (just under the diaphragm) and then move slowly up to the heart area. Acknowledge the feelings and emotions that are coming up and allow any negative thoughts to drift away. Slowly on each breath let your resourceful and positive energy flow in. If you feel concerned, stressed or anxious, focus on more helpful thoughts such as generosity, compassion and acceptance to flow from your gut and heart.

Practising this exercise, where you move from mindfulness and gradual acceptance to compassion and resourcefulness, helps you to put aside intrusions and focus entirely on the person you are supporting and their landscape, co-creating a particular transformative energy flow. It is paying respectful attention to the body movements, the sighs, the breathing and the voice tone of the individuals whatever their background. This allows access to your own intuition and to trust that what arises in the session is there for a reason. Expectation and preconceived ideas about how the session should go are left at the door. You are patient and able to allow for the emergence of what comes.

Empathy or Intrusion?

This can be challenging when the individual brings situations you can identify with. It is useful to remember that no two people ever feel or experience the same issues in quite the same way. It is at these times you need to refrain from entering into the content of the session and remain open to what unfolds. You will also notice that long after the sessions this transformative heartfelt relationship is carried further. All parties are better able to reflect on their own learning and take away new understanding of their situations or issues. Only when nurturing this special connection, keeping out your own ego and intrusive thoughts, can your support of others be truly effective.

The practice of mindfulness is one way you can increase awareness of what is present and to be non-judgmental in sessions. The term mindfulness in Theravada Buddhism is described as Satipathana – *sati* being the element of awareness and *pathana* the element of keeping present.

So how do you maintain heartfelt presence and rekindle the spirit of transformation?

A case study of true presence and personal mindfulness in action

I lived in Switzerland for 14 years from 1972 to 1986. In Switzerland high in the mountains there are incredibly agile mountain goats. They climb in crevices and along ridges that seem impossible to those gazing from below. Many people are unable to see them as they are so far away and so well camouflaged. There are also tiny deer leaping from rock to rock and grazing on the rich grass far away from human habitation. Marmots are also hiding in the undergrowth so shy that people often do not realise they exist.

There are, however, people who have no trouble hearing and seeing these creatures. The mountain people have trained themselves to practise a kind of mindful stillness from within. They are so aware of their own body, presence and surroundings they are able to see and hear with a sharpness so elusive to others. It is this kind of stillness and acute connection with the heart of nature that creates this special bond. If we just take the time to listen and observe, the energy of nature and all it offers will reveal itself and enrich your soul.

I was fortunate in that my father-in-law was a Swiss mountain guide. From the first moment I met him I noticed how he observed and listened attentively to anyone who spoke to him. He responded to the present moment with a profound sense of calm and deep awareness. He seemed to know instinctively what you needed without asking. If you were sad or happy, needed space or company, he would know and with few words was able to convey his love and quiet presence when needed.

He took us to the mountains on many occasions and his connectedness with nature was astounding. I remember feeling frustrated when I was unable to see and hear what he so easily saw and heard. Animals in the shady crevices, tiny mountain flowers, birds high in the sky, trickling water – he had no better hearing or sight, just mindful presence and oneness with all that surrounded him. Slowly I dropped my *wanting* to see and I became still and curious with *less expectation*. I saw a tiny movement. Quietly I observed emotions in my body, began breathing from my heart and noticed my surroundings, just as they were and not as I had imagined. Images, sensations, feelings and sounds all began to have a clarity I had not known before.

I began to discover a real moment to moment awareness of how everything was connected. It was a realisation that all was as it needed to be, in that particular space and time. It was fascinating to realise that aspects of my own way of being and cultural experience had obscured what I felt, saw and heard.

How do you stay mindful and go deeper into the heart and soul of one-to-one sessions?

How often do you feel the need to respond to the pain or challenge of your individuals and in so doing intrude on *their* own way of being and coping? In this way our individuals are interrupted in their own thought process. This can be prevented by increasing awareness of how you are sitting with your individuals/patients. There is a need to be still, relaxed and with hearts and minds open to whatever turns up.

Reflect beforehand on your cultural influencers, racial bias, body language and gestures, noticing how they fit with your words and emotions. It is this quality of attention that shows respect for all and allows for an unconditional positive space for individuals to explore and grow safely.

In this state you notice and understand better the intricacies and often multi-layered relationships involved. When you pay heartfelt attention and are present in the 'now' of the session you can support individuals to clarify their understanding of those sometimes very complex relationships and contexts.

It is the quiet and respectful attention you feel when listening to a wonderful musical performance. The kind of tingle that goes up the spine when the music fills your soul, and the sound enables your heart and mind to soar to unknown heights. When you consider all that individuals bring to the sessions and how present with them you need to be, it is helpful to remember those times when your heart has also been still and attentive. To recall those moments that have touched your heart and allowed you to go deeper to listen to the rhythm of the soul.

A quote from Eckhart Tolle in *The Power of Now* illustrates true presence. He says if you "remove time from the mind – it stops." In essence, he is saying that being present in the now is all you need to still your thoughts. The kind of stillness in unknown territory that captures the brief moments that are so vital and empowering in your work with others.

The use of voice and body

Being present also means paying calm attention to your voice and gestures (which in some cultures may not be appropriate). The voice is an essential part of who we are and how we express ourselves. The stress you put on words and the specific intonation can reveal so much about the intention of the speaker. There are a variety of ways to say, "What exactly do you value most about this situation?" or "When might you take a decision?" Your voice can be gentle and curious or have specific emphasis on "What/When" or on "you" in either question.

Sometimes the stress or intonation is unconscious, and feelings or opinions show through even though you may not realise it. Neutral tone and calm inquiry enable the listener to decide for themselves where to put the emphasis or intonation. This is where Clean Language methodology is so appropriate as it slows the pace and is highly respectful of the individual's world view and cultural background. It purely centres on individual information, phrases and encourages self-empowerment.

Gestures and non-verbal clues mirror your innermost thoughts. Your gestures give away what you really feel and so paying attention to them in the here and now can help you to relax and become grounded and centred.

Top Tips to create presence and mindfulness

1. Pay attention to your breathing from the diaphragm and heart.

2. Align your head, heart and gut to feel balanced and grounded.

3. Picture a calm peaceful scene and return frequently to it.

4. Create heartfelt positive and calm energy for your individuals.

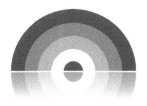

CHAPTER 3

GROUND YOURSELF IN TIMES OF CHAOS

Aga Kehinde

This chapter focuses on the importance of grounding and how to ground yourself into the present situation to restore mental focus when facing challenging times. This is important in the cycle of empowerment because it creates the critical awareness of reality. You are mindful, present and empowered to move forward.

We all have skills and tools we have used in the past to overcome life challenges and obstacles. However, sometimes we may find ourselves facing something that feels stronger and almost impossible to overcome.

Working under pressure in challenging times

Living and caring for others in the current climate is more stressful than ever before. Every day you are likely to face a range of stressors including exposure to trauma, moral injury, workplace stress and home pressure. Adding to what is already a stress-inducing environment, you may now be looking at the real threats of losing your health or (with the recent pandemic) even your life.

Dealing with the unexpected may bring feelings of anxiety surrounding the uncertainty, stress, worry, fear of the unknown, fear of the future, obsessing about the past, inability to think straight or act normally. These all affect work and relationships. This can also have an impact on health, sleep and eating habits or paralyse your thoughts. If you are a healthcare worker or facing challenging times, I am sure you recognise those feelings. Taking care of others while facing exceptional challenges brings a significant worry about the impact this may have on you and your individuals or patients.

Facing the current challenge of a global pandemic may take you out of your comfort zone to a very unstable territory. You may feel out of control and be unable to predict the outcomes. You may also experience a lack or overload of information and witness morally challenging processes.

Daily exposure to stressful conditions may cause you a stress injury or moral trauma which may possibly even lead to post-traumatic stress disorder in the future. When you find yourself in a constant state of high stress and anxiety it can make you feel detached or disassociated, almost like your experiences do not seem real.

Coping strategies from personal experience

This is the time to tune into tools and techniques that I have personally used for many years when working with patients facing life-changing situations. These are strategies that will allow me to restore the order, get rid of the overwhelming fear and anxiety and move mindfully to a safe space. They deactivate fight and flight response and allow me to think clearly. Only then do I start to create personal health and wellbeing strategies. Establishing order externally and internally is paramount to mental health and wellbeing.

Grounding is the number one technique that immediately connects you to the present moment; it reconnects you to reality. Grounding skills can be useful in managing overwhelming feelings like fear or anxiety and help you to regain mental focus.

Understanding the stress response

When facing a threat, real or not, our body naturally switches to an automatic survival mechanism, a state of response called fight, flight or freeze, which prepares us to either fight for survival or run away when threatened.

This process starts from the signal (information we hear and see) being sent to the amygdala. This is the part of our brain responsible for emotional processing, where the information is processed, interpreted and a signal sent to the hypothalamus.

The hypothalamus is the command centre part of our brain and communicates with the rest of the body through the autonomic nervous system. When the amygdala sends the distress signal to the hypothalamus, the sympathetic nervous system is activated and the body's automatic response is immediately activated. All the physical changes in our body are regulated by the sympathetic nervous system and hormones such as cortisol, adrenaline and testosterone. We have no conscious control over these processes.

This automatic body response instigates a cascade of dramatic physical changes like increased heart rate, raised blood pressure and breathing rate. The response is designed to give us an energy burst and strength. When the moment of danger is over, we should naturally return back to a natural, relaxed state.

With the fight and flight response we are wired for action, and when the threat is not real but more a continuum of the anxiety mode, we are using an extremely high amount of energy and body resources. It is vital for our physical and mental wellbeing to move from the stress response to relaxed state as quickly and as often as possible.

Grounding techniques

Many people when in a fight or flight response find it difficult to stop these processes which may lead to stress, overload and injury. Grounding techniques are very useful to bring us back to the relaxed state quickly and effectively.

There are many different grounding techniques that I have been using over the years and each of them is using a slightly different approach:

1. Somatic techniques – using your senses: touch, vision, movement, sound or breathing

2. Cognitive techniques – using mental distraction to redirect the attention away from the anxious feelings

3. Comfort or soothing techniques – using positive anchors (memories)

I would like to introduce you to a technique that combines multiple elements from the list above; it's fast, effective and has long-lasting results.

Emotional Freedom Techniques – the fast and effective way to ground yourself

Emotional Freedom Techniques (EFT) is an evidence-based tool known as *tapping* as it involves gentle tapping on the particular parts of the body. It is described sometimes as a psychological acupuncture as the tapping points are located on the same meridians that are used in the traditional acupuncture.

"Acupoint tapping sends signals directly to the stress centres of the mid-brain, not mediated by the frontal lobes (the thinking part, active in talk therapy)." Dr Dawson Church

EFT is used to change negative feelings rapidly, reduce stress and negative self-limiting thoughts. EFT is easy to learn. You can self-administer EFT at any time. It combines elements of mindfulness, exposure therapy, acceptance and positive affirmation with somatic elements (tapping on the body itself).

"EFT is a true mind-body approach in that it includes direct interventions at the level of the body, it changes brain activity very rapidly and it has special advantages in quickly and permanently shifting outdated emotional learnings." Dr Peta Stapleton

In my experience, using EFT will not only allow you to reduce stress immediately but will also allow you to soothe past memories that may have contributed to the intensity of your current stress response. EFT simultaneously accesses stress at physical and emotional levels.

"EFT gives you the best of both worlds, body and mind, like getting a massage during a psychotherapy session." Dr Dawson Church

Basic technique for grounding using tapping

When you find yourself in a distressing state you can use this basic technique.

Start by focusing on the negative emotion: a fear, anxiety, worry, sadness, anything that is bothering you. Rate this distress or discomfort on a scale 0 to 10 (zero being no distress and 10 extreme distress). This is a SUDS score (Subjective Units of Distress).

To maintain a mental focus (staying mindful, in the present moment) you need to set up the statement. You capture your problem in this statement and will repeat this statement three to four times while gently tapping on the side of your hand below your little finger – see Figure 3.

"Even though I am... (insert your problem/feeling)... I accept how I feel."

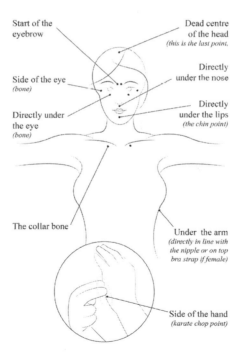

Start of the eyebrow

Dead centre
of the head
(this is the last point.

Side of the eye
(bone)

Directly
under the nose

Directly under
the eye
(bone)

Directly
under the lips
(the chin point)

The collar bone

Under the arm
*(directly in line with
the nipple or on top
bra strap if female)*

Side of the hand
(karate chop point)

Figure 3: Schematic representation of EFT tapping points

Next step is to tap seven or eight times on the eight points on your body (see Figure 3) while repeating a short reminding phrase to make sure your mind is engaged.

The reminding phrase is a shorter version of your set-up statement, focusing only on the feeling, eg:

"stressed"

"anxious"

"worried"

Then you take a deep breath and re-rate the score using a SUDS.

Tapping on these meridian points – while concentrating on accepting and resolving the negative emotion – allows us to quickly restore a balanced state. We are mindfully acknowledging the state we are in. We use tapping and breathing with compassionate acceptance and positive affirmation which immediately calms us down.

Tapping is simple, painless and empowering. It can be learned by anyone and you can apply it to yourself, whenever you want and wherever you are. Most importantly, tapping gives you the power to manage your own stress and anxieties in a matter of minutes and its lasting effect will restore control for the moment and the future.

Some techniques to help grounding:

1. Identify the taste in your mouth and describe it

2. Identify three sources of sound – start from the loudest one

3. Notice three things you can see, describe what you see in your mind

Top Tips

1. Learn how to tap and start to practise right away.

2. Tap on a daily basis so you create the habit of turning to tapping when the stressful situation arises.

3. Take a deep calming breath between each tapping point.

4. Tap as long as you need to bring the score number to 0 or 1.

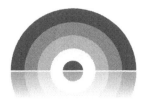

CHAPTER 4

POSSIBILITIES OF USING OUR BODIES TO EMPOWER US

Amanda White

"Our bodies change our minds, our minds change our behaviour and our behaviour changes our outcomes." Amy Cuddy

There is no doubt that we are living through challenging times. It is tempting (particularly for those in caring professions) to focus outwardly, constantly putting others first and ignoring our own needs. Particularly in the western world, there is a focus on what we think, do or say. We quite often ignore the impact our bodies and the way we show up has on our emotions, how others experience us, how we experience ourselves, our achievements and wellbeing. This chapter will focus on your physical presence, what your body tells you about how you can use these to contribute to your overall wellbeing and your impact on others.

You most likely know your health is greatly influenced by the balance between your physical and emotional wellbeing. Nevertheless, it is easy to focus on practical demands – like earning a living, looking after your family and colleagues, keeping appointments. All this, in addition to handling the constant bombardment of news or social media and generally cramming as much as possible into every day. If you neglect either your physical or emotional wellbeing you are quickly in trouble. At best you'll perform less well and fail to fulfil your potential; at worst you'll make yourself ill. It's important to take time to consider how you are coping with these conflicting pressures.

Mind Body Balance

Your body, emotions, and the language you use are strongly interconnected and you are healthiest when all three are in balance. Becoming aware of this balance in your own body and mind is the first step towards empowerment (see Cycle of Empowerment – Figure 1, Chapter 1). If you find ways to take stock regularly, you give yourself opportunities to intervene and redress the balance. This might mean finding enjoyable ways to exercise to release tension and generate endorphins, eating healthily to keep nourished and energised with a strong immune system as you'll read in more detail in other chapters. It might also mean connecting with positive people who contribute to your happiness, developing regular practices such as mindfulness, meditation or yoga, carving out 'me time' to read a book or do something fun or creative.

If you are lucky enough to be fundamentally healthy, this approach can achieve and maintain a good balance. Life, however, is rarely that simple. Achieving balance can be quite a struggle. Maybe you succumb to physical or mental illness out of the blue. You may become overstretched to the point that your health suffers, or you experience a breakdown of some sort. One thing is certain: your body will stop you one way or another when things become too much. Everyone has different levels of resilience. By being alert to your personal warning signs, you can step in to redress your balance before serious physical or emotional problems take over. Those early warning signs are different for each individual.

What are your signs – headaches, stomach upsets, dry mouth, tense muscles in your shoulders or neck, frequent minor illness, palpitations, brain fog or unusual levels of irritability? Whatever they may be, ignore them at your peril! It may feel heroic to work hard, ignoring the signs your body is frantically sending. Working yourself into the ground, however, helps nobody – how can you hope to care for others if you cannot care for yourself? Instead, notice any warnings your body is sending and treat them as an opportunity to evaluate how you are coping and motivate you to do what you need to find balance.

What part does your body play in your wellbeing?

If you ignore the signs your body is sending until too late, you may become ill. What may be possible if you become aware of and highly attuned to your physical *and* emotional needs? You are far more likely to achieve balance, remain well and therefore serve yourself and others more effectively.

A good place to start cultivating greater self-awareness is developing a regular practice to find your neutral zone – to 'ground' or 'centre' yourself. This might be achieved through meditation, mindfulness, or simply taking a few moments at a regular time each day. Try this:

- Find a quiet undisturbed place, close your eyes, breathe deeply, bring your attention inwards and down, feet stable on the ground

- Notice how you feel, any emotions or physical sensations you are experiencing and notice how these exist in your body

- Try not to judge your feelings, let them go and bring yourself to a calm place wherever it feels natural – this could be focused on your stomach or chest; it need not take long and is helpful

With practice, a quick grounding meditation can support you before tackling something challenging, making you fully present and able to cope with whatever life may throw at you. Becoming familiar with how it feels to be grounded makes it easier to notice your body and emotions when you are off balance.

Body, mood and intentions

Your body posture is directly connected with the emotions you feel; you can see someone's emotional state just by observing their physical posture and people can see that in you too. You can often tell if someone is calm, angry, excited or disappointed just by looking at the way they hold themselves. A change in your mood is reflected in your body. This works the other way around too. By changing your physical posture, it is possible to influence your mood. This provides you with exciting possibilities.

The way you hold yourself in your body impacts your mood. In turn, your mood determines your possible actions and influences what you can achieve... or not. By taking responsibility for your mood, you can be an active participant in the general mood of those around you. Moods are contagious – if you can manage your own mood, you can positively influence others.

Typical examples – changing your energy

Let's take four broad situations where you can use your body to generate a mood that will help you be successful. Once you are empowered to take control of your own body, you will be well equipped to help your clients do the same. Practising this yourself will enable you to guide your clients through a similar practice. The first situation would be when you want to build a relationship quickly or connect deeply with someone – perhaps they are upset, nervous or don't trust you yet. Rather than allow their mood to impact you, you can use your body to generate trust. This would involve an open posture with relaxed shoulders, arms and hands. You might be facing or at a slight angle to the other person (preferably without obstacles between you). You'll be breathing evenly and slowly, maintaining good eye contact, smiling, nodding and actively listening to them. Your energy will be inviting the person towards you.

Another time, you might need to be very action oriented to achieve something quickly and efficiently. Perhaps people around you do not have the same sense of urgency as you, so need to be motivated. If you use your body, moving quickly and purposefully, standing tall and oozing confidence, people are more likely to follow your lead. You will be leaning forward, eyes focused, breathing evenly at a moderate or fast pace. Your energy will be forward. Putting your body in this pattern will help you remain emotionally focused and you will get that important thing done, bringing others along with you.

There may well be times where you need to keep calm when all around you are panicking. The more stable you appear in your body, the more stable you will feel emotionally and the better you will be able to calm yourself and others. It will be helpful to be very grounded, to have your feet solid on the floor with an upright posture. You'll be breathing evenly at a moderate to slow pace – you can certainly calm your own nervous system by taking a few deep breaths. Your eyes will be taking in a broad view and your expression is likely to be neutral. So, if you're feeling distracted or beginning to panic, think about putting your body into this very stable state – fake it till you make it!

Alternatively, you may want to kick back and be adventurous or spontaneous – perhaps to generate ideas, lighten up an atmosphere or play with a child or pet. Even if you're exhausted and don't feel very light-hearted, you can use your body to influence your mood. Try moving around lightly and quickly, maybe on tiptoe or even dancing. You are likely to be smiling, laughing – your expression changing rapidly, your eyes darting all over the place, your energy moving outwards and back to your centre. Especially at times of stress and pressure, developing an ability to generate lightness is a valuable skill.

Consider where you are most naturally comfortable. Are you naturally predisposed to be open, action oriented, stable, or light-hearted? Which of these feels less comfortable for you? Those are the ones to practise, to achieve balance and versatility. Particularly when you are pressurised and challenged, you may spend your working day being serious, focused and trying to generate stability. For those of us working in organisations, when you have a break with your team (or finally go home) you need to lighten up and have some fun to redress the balance. Think about when it would help you to be a bit more open, focused, calm or light-hearted and practise putting your body into the right positions to generate the appropriate emotion, positively impacting yourself and others.

With practice, achieving the versatility to switch comfortably between moods by using your body is empowering. You will have the confidence that you can use your body to support you in dealing with the widest possible range of situations with ease. Being keenly in tune with your body is valuable. It empowers you to ensure you are physically and emotionally healthy, which in turn enables you to support others effectively.

Top Tips

1. Bring regular focus to your physical and emotional state – notice your breathing and muscular tensions. Breathe deeply and quietly, scan from feet to head – what happened?

2. Practise using your body to support your intentions – practise openness, focus, stability and lightness and notice their impact on you and other people.

3. Notice other people's bodies – do they provide insight into how they are feeling?

4. Explore using your body in new ways (eg dancing, running, quietly meditating) – see how you feel and what possibilities arise.

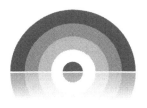

CHAPTER 5

PERSPECTIVES ON BUILDING A HEALTHY IMMUNE SYSTEM

Victoria Hamilton

Why does your immune system matter for health and wellbeing?

The immune system is fundamental to the body as it protects you from infectious diseases such as viruses and bacteria. It also provides you with ongoing protection from non-transmissible diseases by screening your cells for damage. This helps to prevent the onset of conditions such as cancer and autoimmune disease. There are two parts of the immune system: a short-term defence system and a long-term quality control unit. These two systems are known as the innate and adaptive immune system respectively. The first line of defence helps to kill foreign pathogens before they cause damage to your body. Cleverly, the secondary immune system's specialised quality control unit allows immune cells to identify whether a particle is a helpful friend or dangerous foe.

The immune system has heightened surveillance systems at your body's mucosal linings, such as the barrier between the gastrointestinal tract and the bloodstream. Any weakness in these barriers will lead to issues in the body as the immune system will not be able to function as effectively. When these systems become impaired and break down, you may not feel at your best and chronic illness may follow.

How do you know if your immune system is malfunctioning?

When your immune system is not functioning optimally, you may be more prone to catching infections such as the common cold or the flu which relate to a decrease in the immune system's defence. Alternatively, symptoms which relate to a defect in the immune system's quality control process may start more subtly. If caught early, you have a better chance of healing the issues without long-term injury to your body.

Some of these symptoms are associated with chronic low-grade systemic inflammation. This is a result of the immune system becoming fired up continually. This stimulation of the immune system is often a result of the interaction of immune cells with an antigen, which is a particle recognised by the immune system as foreign (using the above terminology, foe). When the immune system is dysfunctional, it may also start to identify your organs and tissues or common food particles as a foe as it is unable to distinguish between the two correctly. As a result, the immune cells can start damaging organs and tissues, leading to chronic disease.

Symptoms of low-grade systemic inflammation include (but are not limited to):

- Fatigue and lack of energy
- Chronic pain, particularly in the muscles, joints or bones
- Headaches
- Dry eyes, mouth or skin
- Difficulty exercising
- Abdominal pain and bloating
- Dark circles under your eyes
- Heat intolerance

Furthermore, you are more likely to suffer from low-grade systemic inflammation in the following cases:

- You have high blood sugar: this may be a result of various factors such as high sugar and refined carbohydrate diet, issues regulating your blood sugar, or dysbiosis in the gastrointestinal tract

(an imbalance of natural bacterial colonies in the gut)

- You are overweight: adipose tissue (fat cells) is itself inflammatory, so having more of it means that you are more likely to have inflammation in your body

- You are not getting enough sleep (less than seven hours per night): when you sleep, your immune system replenishes and restores; if you are not getting enough, your immune system is more likely to be impaired, leading to systemic inflammation

Checking in with your body periodically and understanding when a symptom you are feeling might require further investigation is fundamental to health empowerment. Keeping a food and symptom journal can help considerably with this. Tracking what you eat and how you feel can provide some great insights. It gives information on your body's trends and what food makes you feel most energised versus those that bring unwanted symptoms. Some functional areas to track are food, energy, pain, exercise, digestion and mood. It is also best to use a scale from say 1-10, which provides a useful tool for comparisons when you are reflecting in your journal.

What triggers your immune system to become unbalanced?

The immune system is reliant on a vast number of nutrients and minerals to work effectively. Food is the predominant source of these compounds, so a healthy digestive system is vital for an optimal functioning immune system. The gut wall houses a phenomenal 70% of the immune system, so if you have issues in your digestive system, you more than likely have a problem with your immune system as well. As Hippocrates infamously said, "All disease starts in the gut," and remarkably, some 2,000 years later we are still exploring this prophecy today.

An essential factor in the immune health of the digestive system is a substance called Secretory IgA (SIgA). IgA is an antibody which is part of the immune system's first line of defence. It is in the mucosal lining of the mouth, respiratory and digestive tract. SigA is secreted in the gastrointestinal tract to protect you from the pathogens found on food. It also helps with quality control, 'tagging' substances which can enter the bloodstream vs those that the immune system should destroy. A low amount of SigA is associated with chronic health problems, as well as allergies and food intolerances.

Helpful commensal bacteria found in the gut induce the production of SigA. Eating foods and taking supplements which strengthen the gut microbiome will improve digestion and immune health overall. To encourage the production of SigA, eat vitamin A-rich foods such as organ meats, and orange and yellow vegetables such as sweet potato and butternut squash. Studies show that supplementing with Saccharomyces boullardii also helps to increase SigA in the gut.

Many other factors cause the immune system to become imbalanced such as lack of sleep, poor nutrition, not enough movement in the day, past trauma, difficulty managing stress, a high toxic load from pollutants in the air and food, and an increased exposure to pathogens such as viruses and bacteria. As a personalised nutritional approach is imperative for health empowerment and progression, it is worth exploring what your triggers might be.

As this is a complex area, it is best to work with a qualified healthcare practitioner to explore your underlying triggers so that you can take steps to personalise your diet and lifestyle. A qualified health practitioner will be able to prepare a health assessment, plot a customised timeline of notable life events, and perform functional testing to understand what the contributing and provoking factors in your health and wellbeing are. True health empowerment is about understanding your own body and what works for you alone.

What practical steps can you take to start living a healthier and happier life?

There are many 'biohacks' that you can start incorporating into your life today to begin on your path to wellness and health empowerment. With the amount of contradicting information on health and wellbeing, and many taking 'Dr Google's' advice, it is hard to know what is best to do to be healthy. However, living a healthy lifestyle is easier than you think. Positive everyday habits are the best way to be healthy long term.

Building a healthy immune system is important for you as a practitioner and for the individuals you work with.

Top Tips

1. Cook at least one meal a day from scratch.

2. Eat the rainbow in colours of vegetables each week: having a list of vegetables categorised by colour which you can check off.

3. Incorporate healthy fats in your diet every day.

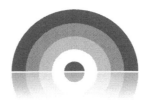

CHAPTER 6

NATURE AND SPIRITUALITY

Sue Jackson and Fiona Stimson

"In every walk with nature one receives far more than he seeks."
John Muir

Sowing the seeds

The world and our experiences of it have changed dramatically in recent times due to the COVID-19 pandemic and the unprecedented measures needed to limit its impact. We have been catapulted into a life of Zoom meetings, staying safe by staying at home and the resultant sense of isolation.

In this chapter we show how the effects of nature, spirituality and the interplay of both impacts positively on our personal wellness, sense of connection and health empowerment. These resources are especially important in challenging personal and global crises.

We are sharing our personal experiences, training and practices as professional coaches. These experiences enrich and empower us in our own personal and professional lives and the individuals we serve. There is a large body of research which evidences much of our experience and you can do a deep dive into this through Google Scholar.

We consider nature as the earth, sky, water and all life: plants, animals and microbes. Spirituality is the quality of being concerned with the human spirit or soul in its widest non-religious context. In our experience, nature and spirituality become intertwined when we feel connected to the natural world.

The benefits of being in and connecting with nature

You can experience, interact with and notice nature in many ways. It can help you to restore and regenerate your resources. It is fundamental to good health.

Walking, sitting, lying in or observing nature raises awareness, creates curiosity, joy, hope and provides a context for reflection. It helps to solve challenges, be creative or simply relax and recuperate. When you experience the Earth's energy it creates a sense of grounding, wholeness and empowerment.

The research evidence on the health benefits of connecting with nature are impressive, from reduced blood pressure to improving focus, memory and energy.

The natural world helps you to recover from the fatigue of your mental concentration by restoring attention. The benefits of the sunlight are important too, it gives you much-needed vitamin D and has associated positive effects on the immune system.

Benefits from nature can also be derived when you look out of a window at greenery or at the sky. If you are unable to physically 'be' in it either through lack of opportunity or health constraints, a found object like a pebble or a photograph of a favourite place can act as an anchor for you to engage with past memories and generate positive emotions and health benefits. Research shows that looking out on nature (as opposed to a brick wall) aids recovery from surgery. Connection with nature is important in the design of healthcare buildings and in communities, for mental and emotional health.

The colours that dominate nature are green and blue. These colours stimulate calm, spaciousness and tranquillity. Research shows that being in both green and blue spaces is beneficial for your wellbeing. Water provides auditory, visual and physiological stimulation. It can help you to unwind, connect and reflect. The negative ions generated by water ground pollution particles, reducing lung irritation and allergies.

Your sensory dance with nature

Your sense of smell is stimulated in the natural environment, for example damp woodland, the smell of honeysuckle or salty air. This can engage memories and be a powerful means of reconnection to the narrative of your life. Using natural scents can benefit your health and relaxation; for example, citrus oils increase attention, lift mood and help balance.

Your sense of touch can be stimulated by walking barefoot in grass, running your fingers through meadow grasses or feeling water running through your fingers. You may also sense the pressure of the atmosphere, which may affect how you think, feel and behave.

The sounds of nature, for example birdsong, bring joy to many; it raises attention levels, curiosity, brings you into the moment and may have a spiritual dimension.

Looking up at the sky both in the day and night helps you take a break from cognitively demanding tasks. It expands your awareness and brings a sense of awe and wonder. It generates calmness, a greater sense of connection and a more expansive sense of perspective. The new study of Skychology (Conway) describes how looking up at the sky enhances your psychological wellbeing and ameliorates physical discomfort.

"Nature nurtures our health; it provides a space of solace in chaos, ease from demands, meaning from confusion and connection for the soul." Sue Jackson

Personal growth through coaching with nature

Nature contact encourages curiosity, enquiry and exploration in the coaching process. We are all different in our relationship with the natural world; for example, you may feel calm or find it difficult to relax. Coaching in nature can support you to learn from the feelings and emotions experienced and begin to find resources in its many benefits.

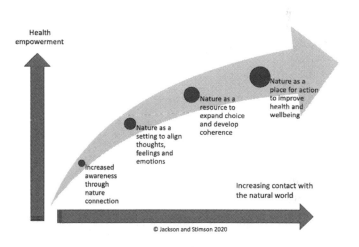

Figure 4: Nature as a resource for health empowerment

Nature creates flow for both the coach and individual. Freer thinking and the space created generates choices from which you, as the individual or coach, can act, review and learn. Nature-based coaching can change your perspective, your behaviours and empower you to care for your wellbeing and health.

Working with individuals, practitioners notice the benefits of greater presence and stronger alignment and relatedness. Mindful breathing and grounding practices in nature support the opening of the self, acceptance and courageous action. As practitioners we experience it as important in our self-compassion and gratitude practices. Natural ecosystems, rhythms and patterns create meaning for us.

The use of metaphor and Clean Language in coaching conversations in nature can help describe something that is going on within in a different way. Nature metaphors stimulate personal and individual thinking, learning and reflections, using for example the stability of trees, the fluidity of and reflections from water. They may relate to the rhythms of nature, for example the ephemeral nature of flowers, leaf fall in autumn, frogspawn, butterflies and the unfurling of ferns in spring.

There are many examples of the personal rewards and health empowerment from coaching in nature. Two illustrations are given below:

The first is an example of a walking coaching session with an individual in London. The individual works as a newly appointed director, struggling to manage the challenges of work, travel and medical treatments. We walked into a large park and on reaching the top of a hill overlooking the city, we stopped and could see the city laid out before us. When prompted with the question, "What are you noticing?" after some time her reply was, "My life is like this city plan, detailed and busy with areas that are like the green spaces, places of quiet and relaxation." After a short silence, she continued, "I need to make those green spaces bigger and more important." This observation and realisation generated a springboard for our continued exploration and determining action which aligned mentally and emotionally with the goals that had emerged for her during this connection to the landscape and nature.

Another powerful experience is a 'Mindful Coach Walk' with the purpose of empowering individuals to manage their health and wellness. Individuals walk in silence, immersing themselves in the sensory experience guided by the coach. On the return walk home, there is a sharing of experiences and learning. It teaches coaches a lot about the challenges people face, their pain and suffering, and offers awareness and motivation for action in the individual. Being with individuals in silence (our coaching presence) in nature can be a source of new insights and transformation. For example, the sharing of silent experiences in the confidential coaching space of the return walk home allows an individual to express their heartfelt self and vulnerabilities, an extremely powerful and rarely gained experience. This has also been successful in small intimate groups where the combination of learning is shared with wonderfully positive outcomes for all to take away.

"The intelligence of nature can transform human consciousness, we can tap into it at any given moment to help nourish and heal our mind, body and soul." Fiona Stimson

Nature, spirituality and coaching

During lockdown, the social distancing, isolation, the trauma of illness and death has resulted for some in loss of connection and sense of common humanity. Spiritual development can help mitigate this as it involves seeking a meaningful connection with something bigger than oneself.

The practice of mindfulness and expanding your awareness takes time and focus. A coach skilled in these practices can support you in this. Once mastered, you can explore perspectives, meaning and loosen boundaries that may have been holding you back in life, resulting in greater ease, flow and a deeper sense of self. In our personal experience, expanded awareness heightens intuition, awe and connection. If you ground feelings such as gratitude, compassion, love and appreciation for yourself and those around you while in this expanded state, then you are more likely to feel content.

Nature has a way of making you aware of time and its passing. More fallow or dormant times are part of the cycle and predictability of the natural world. You can align yourself with its rhythms. Nature reminds us we are human and may hold treasured memories. It can be comforting and support your spiritual wellness when all around you may be uncertain and chaotic transition. In the spring lockdown of the northern hemisphere due to the pandemic, engaging with emergent life and growth and the hope, wonder and reassurance it provided was an empowering resource.

The impermanence of clouds reminds us all to be in the moment and that any attempt to hold on to things that are external is not possible. Cloud watching and noticing can provide you with a useful practice for acceptance and letting go of rumination and worries.

Being with or in nature allows you the time and space to step back from whatever else is going on in your life. It enables you to restore balance, acknowledge what you may be thinking or feeling. Being immersed in nature is a way to reduce anxieties and worries, encourage the flow of beneficial hormones, restoring your mental and physiological wellness.

Coaching with nature and spirituality engages you in the health empowerment cycle. It raises your awareness to make choices in ways that align with the internal and external motivations that are critical to you. Within this framework you can then make proactive and sustainable changes aligned with your values and reflect on the effect of these.

During the first wave of the coronavirus pandemic many people, us included, gained solace from our connection with nature. It supported our mental, emotional, spiritual and physical health. Nature helps us realise that we are integrated with the living world and wider Universe and not separate from it. This value we placed on the natural world has been a way for the population to reflect on the damage to our climate and natural environment caused by our behaviours and economic systems. It has opened our thinking and public discussion to the benefits and imminent need to adopt pro-environmental behaviours. Health and the Environment are two of the most important UN Global Goals for Sustainable Development.

Setting the seed

Nature and the links into spirituality it produces provide us, our communities and our world with a myriad of resources for our health, wellbeing and the development of our common humanity. Nature supports our sense of empowerment by increasing our awareness, using information that is shared or we discover, and learning new ways to be in and respond to the natural world.

Coaching in nature is a context for transformation for us and the individuals we work with. It creates flow and authenticity through exploration of a deeper sense of who we truly are. It helps us develop our sense of coherence and promotes our health. We find meaning in nature's rhythms, beauty and growth. It is a free source of wisdom and learning and a place for physical activity.

When engaging with the natural world in our lives and our coaching, we are only too aware of the urgent need to value, respect and conserve it.

Top Tips

1. Organise your spaces to maximise views of nature, indoor plants and found treasures, particularly if you are ill, stressed, or anxious.

2. Take a daily short walk – you benefit from the movement, natural light and the spiritual connection of engaging with nature.

3. Practise mindfulness in nature – notice the finer details, sights, sounds, smells and feelings whilst intermittently focusing on your natural breathing.

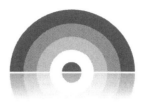

PART 2:
INFORMATION

In this section you are led down a second exciting path of discovery and learning. You will enhance your knowledge of how to increase empowerment through enabling personal leadership. By working with the narrative of your individuals, you develop shared decision making and apply simple measures of health and wellbeing. You will gain insights into how to create empathy and enhance practitioner–patient relationships. You will be encouraged to delve into essential breathwork, emotion regulation, and learn about biofeedback. By using this information, you will also increase your overall knowledge and awareness of essential health and wellness strategies for a sustainable healthy lifestyle.

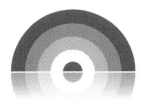

CHAPTER 7

COACHING FOR PERSONAL LEADERSHIP: AN ESSENTIAL APPROACH FOR HEALTH IN TIMES OF CHANGE AND UNCERTAINTY

Andrew A Parsons and Sue Jackson

"Change is the only constant." Heraclitus

Supporting people through change is a very personal and human-centric experience, which may take the form of dialogue with a friend, family member, or engaging with a professional skilled in this process. Change occurs in all parts of our lives: societal (eg a global pandemic), organisational (eg business restructuring), professional (eg promotion), relational (eg divorce) or personal (eg receiving a life-changing medical diagnosis). We experience a range of different perspectives, options, challenges and emotions in all changes as we move from the old and familiar to the new and unfamiliar, through uncertain territory.

Changes are events and transitions are the internal psychological reorientation processes that we go through when we experience change (Bridges, 1980). Bridges' Model of Transition has three key stages The first, 'the ending', involves us being with the sense of loss and letting go of what has been or how we imagined our life would be. The second phase is the 'neutral zone' where everything seems disorientated, up for grabs and brings with it both discomfort as life is neither familiar nor the new way and possibilities as we move to consider options to create a different life. The third stage is the phase of new beginnings, where we start to develop and adapt to our new identity and perspectives. In this, we experience new energy, utilise our resources and discover the sense of purpose that makes us feel more orientated in the present and able to navigate our challenges.

Maintaining health through transitions can be demanding. Stress, anxieties and other heightened emotional responses can have immediate and long-term consequences. There is a key role for coaching practitioners to support the development of personal leadership behaviours with individuals so that they embrace transition and uncertainty with a greater sense of empowerment. For the purpose of this chapter, we define personal leadership as the ability to lead oneself and others to develop awareness and access resources for optimal health.

Personal leadership development: health empowerment in change

Figure 5 below provides an overview of the areas of collaborative coaching enquiry to develop personal leadership. The emerging dialogue between the coach practitioner and the individual explores the latter's attitudes, values, beliefs and personal behaviours which impact on their health and wellbeing. Wellbeing can be defined as the balance point between an individual's resource pool and the challenges faced. An individual's resource pool is enhanced by engaging with the five keys to wellbeing (New Economics Foundation): take notice, connect, give, be active and keep learning.

This develops cognitive strategies and skills, awareness (mindful practice), leadership of self and others, and enables critical and active participation for maintaining health, especially in times of change and uncertainty.

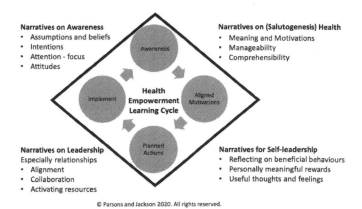

Narratives on Awareness
- Assumptions and beliefs
- Intentions
- Attention - focus
- Attitudes

Narratives on (Salutogenesis) Health
- Meaning and Motivations
- Manageability
- Comprehensibility

Health Empowerment Learning Cycle

Awareness
Aligned Motivations
Implement
Planned Actions

Narratives on Leadership
Especially relationships
- Alignment
- Collaboration
- Activating resources

Narratives for Self-leadership
- Reflecting on beneficial behaviours
- Personally meaningful rewards
- Useful thoughts and feelings

Figure 5: Collaborative coaching enquiry: a Narrative Framework for exploring emergent goals to develop personal leadership

As discovered in Chapter 1, the three core elements in coaching for health empowerment are awareness, information and learning. This Personal Leadership Framework uses the cycle of empowerment for learning and supports the emergence of goals and motivation for action through collaborative dialogue. The development of cognitive strategies combined with the skills of awareness and leadership enables critical and active participation in transitioning to new beginnings. As coach practitioners, bringing these principles, strategies and behaviours into our own lives we are more able to support the development of others. Our narrative coaching approach is a Third Generation approach as described by Reinhard Stelter.

We will expand below on each of the cornerstones of the Coaching for Personal Framework to provide guidance and useful information for personal learning and empowerment and in the coaching process.

Awareness

Awareness can support changes in attitudes, beliefs and behaviours. It requires us to engage our intention towards, attention on and adopt attitudes that promote mindful practice. Building the skills of mindfulness changes the ways in which our brains function, developing heightened noticing, greater adaptability and coping skills. Practitioners can engage with Kabat-Zinn's Attitudinal Foundations to Mindfulness and use exercises to build the skills of attention and awareness for themselves and with individuals – for example, using nature, biofeedback and emotions. These resources contribute to our information, learning, presence, rich coaching dialogue and opportunities for growth.

Being healthy - salutogenesis

Creating a state of 'good health' focuses on both the reduction of health risks and the promotion of resources to maintain and improve health. To stay healthy, you benefit from having belief in your capacity to cope in adapting and responding to the events in your life. This way of thinking about health is called salutogenesis and was first introduced by the medical sociologist Aaron Antonovsky in the 1970s-1980s (see further reading).

Saluto (*health*) genesis (*promotion*) is an approach to understanding the complex relationship between stress, health, coping and wellbeing along the continuum between good health and dis-ease. When you are facing a 'stressor', the resulting 'tension' that occurs can either be overcome by your health promoting (salutogenic) resources or eventually lead to breakdown, pathogenesis and dis-ease. Antonovsky termed the ability of individuals to manage their health continuum a "sense of coherence (SOC)" which he explained as the *"perception of an individual on the stimuli bombarding him."*

If you have a strong SOC and encounter challenges, you utilise your available resources to become motivated to cope (meaningfulness) in ways that make sense to you. You can see how things fit together for you in your situation (comprehensibility) and believe you have enough resources to cope, even if you do not feel in overall control (manageability). Anotonovksy's approach transcends cultural boundaries and at the same time it is very personal to you. It provides a framework for learning through our experiences that *'promotes health'* when you are faced with the stressors and tensions of life.

Leading myself: strategies for creating active participation

In parallel with the emergence of salutogenesis the concept of self-leadership has developed in the scientific literature over the last 30 years. It is defined as the ability to influence oneself to perform activities and tasks. Self-leadership involves cognitive processes (useful thoughts and feelings), aligning motivations (assessing what needs to be done), how it is to be done and what's important about its completion. We consider personal leadership as a crucial component for empowerment and a useful resource to promote health.

There are three key strategies that promote self-leadership that can be explored in coaching:

1. Developing useful cognitions

Coaching is an ideal environment to explore your thinking, feelings, narratives, beliefs and assumptions that facilitate action. In a rapidly changing situation with high uncertainty, focusing attention in the present leads to greater capacity for health-promoting thoughts regarding the manageability, comprehension and meaning in the current situation.

2. Changes in behaviour

Coaching generates greater awareness through self-reflection, feedback and review of specific actions, behaviours or habits that may be modified to enhance the achievement of individuals' emergent goals. This is an iterative learning process generated through the coaching conversations.

3. Focus on natural rewards (personally meaningful, see below)

Meaning and motivation are important for action. They can be the drive for change, for growth or adaptation. Coaching to support you to align your intrinsic or autonomous motivations and to develop positive perceptions of unappealing tasks can create your drive for sustainable action. These natural rewards can create a sense of meaning or purpose and are a salutogenic resource (providing meaningfulness).

Self-determination theory provides a framework for coaches and other professionals to explore motivations and provides a deeper understanding of natural rewards. The building blocks of self-determination – autonomy, relatedness and competence – are essential for the development of 'self' in an active and dynamic learning process, which supports you to adapt and progress. As coaching practitioners our aim is to satisfy these needs so that you optimise your development. You develop skills (competence) and your own plans of action (autonomy) in a professional relationship that is supportive, trusting and where you feel safe and understood (relatedness). In our coaching we can work with you in this way if you have long-term medical conditions and/or challenging health diagnoses by taking into account the limits imposed by your diagnosis and treatment.

One key aspect of the self-determination theory is the impact of different motivations on our behaviours. Our motivations from within, which are aligned with our concept of self, are termed intrinsic, and those driven by external factors, extrinsic. Extrinsic motivations split into two broad groups termed controlled or autonomous. Controlled motivations drive our behaviours because we feel that we should act because of a social expectation. Autonomous motivations differ in that they drive our behaviour, being something either we like to do or brings us personal value. These 'natural rewards' are an important part of our development of self-leadership strategies.

Some tools are available in the resources section of this book to support these meaningful conversations. These include reflective questions regarding the five behaviours of wellbeing, a link to Neil's Wheel (a tool to facilitate meaningful conversations), and the presence pyramid (a framework to develop strategies regarding self-management within your social environment).

Leading us: strategies for reciprocal participation

Leadership creates alignment, motivation and direction and is generally considered in the context of professional activities. However, we all have an opportunity to use leadership skills in other aspects of our lives, for example our own health. The majority of people live in relationships with their families, friends, work colleagues and communities. Freire defined empowerment as involving 'active participation' to create alignment, direction and motivation towards our common goals, therefore it is an active reciprocal exchange.

Coaching conversations support learning by exploring the narratives regarding the core elements of 'leading others' (Figure 1), namely alignment, collaboration and finding resources. Through the coaching exploration, we, as practitioners, find ways for you to be in sync with other people you can influence and find ways to act that are mutually beneficial.

Conclusion

In times of uncertainty and change when goals are still evolving, a narrative coaching process with its focus on awareness, health, self-leadership and collaboration creates a means by which the new beginning and goals can emerge to allow you to move towards your new and empowered reality.

As coaching practitioners, exploring your narratives with you in the collaborative coaching process creates learning opportunities to manage transitions and optimise health and wellness.

Top Tips

1. Listen to your stories – use what is useful now to shift the narrative towards your future.

2. Bring your attention to what is meaningful now – place your energy to develop and align with your level of motivation.

3. Take time to identify all the resources available to you – skills, experience, strengths, values, people and anything 'outside the box'.

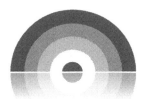

CHAPTER 8

PATIENT-CENTRED CARE: ENHANCING EMPOWERMENT THROUGH SHARED DECISION MAKING

Silvia Mirandola

The healthcare system is changing

Medicine has become increasingly complex and it is evolving at a very rapid pace, thus requiring new skills and new processes for delivering high-quality healthcare services. Mark Britnell, chairman of KPMG's Global Health Practice, says, *"Healthcare needs to move from Transactional (doing things better) to Transformational (doing better things)."*

Artificial intelligence (AI) and related technologies are increasingly prevalent in business and society and are beginning to be applied to healthcare. In the near future, doctors are likely to increase their use of AI and machine learning devices to improve precision in diagnosis and in therapy regimens.

While computers may support diagnosis, the human touch will be important. The relational skills that create empowerment for the individual such as empathy, listening and collaboration will be needed. The results that can be obtained (the *what)* depends not only by the processes applied (the *how)* but on the quality of the relationship (the *who*) between patient and clinician and by the intention and attention that the doctor addresses during the encounter.

The quality of the relationship between caregiver and patient is the single most important determinant of effective medical intervention. In a recent Italian survey on success factors in healthcare, results highlight that one of the main factors is the relationship between patient and physician. Without a balanced patient-physician relationship, no healthcare system can work properly.

This kind of 'relationship-caring' could be the turning point for shifting the health system from ego-system, which addresses our needs, to eco-system, the awareness of the system and the connection and relationships of its components.

Patient-centred care and empowerment

From doing things 'to' the patient... to doing things 'with' the patient

Chronic diseases are seen as a sustainability challenge for European health systems in terms that include its financing, its organisation and the delivery of services. Supporting people with chronic diseases and long-term conditions requires a fundamental shift from the disease-centred to patient- and family-centred approach. This attitudinal shift also requires the combination of patient self-management with integration to a multidisciplinary integrated professional team.

It is important to remember that patients are experts in their own lived experience. Their perspective on their medical condition/disease and their optimal care is unique and is a resource to be utilised. Their active participation in the transformation of their world (empowerment) requires their active involvement at every level in the health system. In the broadest sense, active patient involvement is needed in policy making and in the co-designing of care services to meet their needs more effectively.

Patient-centred care is defined as: *'Providing care that is respectful of and responsive to individual patient preferences, need, and values, and ensuring that patient values guide all clinical decisions.'*

The principles of patient-centred healthcare have been defined and include:

1. Respect for patients' unique needs, preferences, autonomy

2. Choice of appropriate treatment option that best fits patients' needs

3. Patient empowerment and involvement in decisions that concern their health

4. Access to safe, high-quality, appropriate services and support

5. Information that is reliable, relevant and understandable

6. Patient involvement in health policy to ensure services are designed with the patient at the centre

Interprofessional collaboration

The complexity of the healthcare system and the escalation of the incidence of chronic diseases requires person-centred healthcare to be provided by a team of diverse professionals. The team objective is to deliver the right care at the right time across the continuum of care. Interprofessional collaboration, including acknowledging the patient as a full member of the team, has been identified by WHO as one of the most promising solutions to improve the patient experience, clinical outcomes and patient safety, thereby transforming the healthcare system.

Interprofessionality is a fundamental concept that can help explain the processes that are required to satisfy the patient's needs.

"Interprofessional collaborative patient-centred practice is one of the most promising solutions to improve the quality of care, the clinical outcomes and the patient safety."

The core characteristics of interprofessionality are:

- continuous interaction
- knowledge sharing to address education and care issues
- patient participation
- adherence to an ethical code of conduct
- integrated collaborative workflow

Healthcare Professionals (HCPs), particularly nurses and clinicians, support the development of a person-centred service through collaborative decision making, where the patient feels they have a voice which is heard by their service providers. Evidence demonstrates that such an interprofessional and collaborative process has significant benefits for all healthcare stakeholders. These benefits include the provision of evidence-based practice, reduced waiting times, the creation of healthy workplaces, the improvement of patient safety and reduction in management and healthcare.

Communication skills such as those used in coaching are essential to ensure this patient-centred approach delivers successful behavioural and clinical outcomes.

Shared Decision Making (SDM)

Effective communication provides understanding of individual intentions and perspectives. It requires information sharing and dialogue, and fosters trust to promote long-term relationships between the patient and clinician. The goal of SDM is to enable patients to make the best preferred decisions with the healthcare team after considering research evidence and experiences in non-emergent or non-life-threatening situations.

SDM is a two-way approach to ignite patients' mastery and accountability in the management of the chronic health condition and in the dialogue with the healthcare provider. It is a key component of patient-centred healthcare and the opposite of clinicians making decisions on behalf of patients. It is a process in which clinicians and patients work together to make decisions, select options, tests, treatments and care plans based on clinical evidence. It takes account of the provider's knowledge and experience while ensuring patient preferences and values are actively considered in balancing risks and expected outcomes. In the context of the empowerment cycle, the SDM process ensures the practitioner and patients are developing critical awareness of information and preferences and ensuring alignment on motivation for action (see Chapter 1). It provides a means by which both parties can be empowered.

There are multiple benefits of SDM for both patient (eg feeling involved), clinician (eg better patient adherence to treatment regimens), their relationship (eg improved trust) and the healthcare system (better outcomes, reduced costs).

Coaches may work directly with HCPs and/or patients to build the skills and confidence to integrate SDM into their practice.

There are different approaches for Shared Decision Making. Here we describe the 3-Talk approach, a three-step process for shared decision making that includes:

1. Team Talk

2. Option Talk

3. Decision Talk

Team Talk

Clinician and patient work as a team to come to the best decision. The clinician makes the patient aware that choice exists and explores the patient's overall goals in relation to their health issue.

Conversation starters:

"Now that we have identified the problem it's time to think about what to do next. I'd like us to make this decision together."

"There is good information about how these treatments differ that I'd like to discuss with you before we decide on an approach that is best for you."

"I'm happy to share my views and help you reach a good decision. Let's work as a team. I am here to support you. Before I do, may I describe the options in more detail?"

Option Talk

This step involves discussing the benefits and risks of the treatment options, so the provider's knowledge about risks and benefits of a treatment and the use of evidence-based decision aids are very important to this step.

Conversation starters:

"Here are some choices we can consider."

"Let me tell you what the research says about the benefits and risks of the medicine/ treatments that you are considering."

"These options will have different implications for you compared to other people, so I want to describe them."

"These tools have been designed to help you to understand your options in more detail."

"What questions do you have?"

"What more information do you need?"

"Is there anything that you don't understand?"

Decision Talk

The clinician is trying to understand what is really important to the patient, what are the issues that are in the back of their mind. Some healthcare providers may not be aware of the outcomes that matter most to patients. In fact, studies have shown that healthcare professionals aren't truly tuned into the things that really matter to patients.

Conversation starters:

"When you think about the possible risks, what matters most to you?"

"As you think about your options, what's important to you?"

"Which of the options fits best with the treatment goals we've discussed?"

"Is there anything that may get in the way of doing this?"

"It's fine to take more time to think about the treatment choices. Would you like some more time, or are you ready to decide?"

"What additional questions do you have for me to help you make your decision?"

"Now that we have had a chance to discuss your treatment options, which treatment do you think is right for you?"

"If you don't feel things are improving, please schedule a follow-up visit so we can plan a different approach."

At the heart of the empowerment approach is seeing the patient-professional relationship as a partnership of equals, as a team focused on common goals where all parties can contribute to reach the goal. This shift from an 'I' perspective to a 'we' perspective is essential to facilitate synergistic outcomes. A healthy 'we' is to foster mutual gain, creating a win-win outcome through cooperation and constructive and transformative dialogue leading to the shift from ego-system to eco-system.

This 3-Talk model developed by Elwyn and colleagues is a practical and effective approach. Coaching skills and competencies will enable the process and provide support for both patients and HCPs in the process.

Top Tips

1. Switch the mindset – from doing things **to** the patient to doing things **with** the patient.

2. Embrace Shared Decision Making (SDM) – it builds trust between patient and clinician, and it makes the patient feel valued and respected.

3. Learn about the 3-Talk approach – it is one of the best models for SDM.

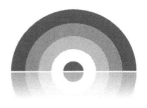

CHAPTER 9

THE DOCTOR'S ROLE IN PATIENT EMPOWERMENT

Enrico Illuminati

"In order to create a learning environment with our patients, doctors and other healthcare professionals need to attend to their attitude towards them."

From the place of 'telling' to 'sharing' our decisions

Since early practice, medicine has taken the form of a science (and an 'art'). Its practitioners have drawn upon specialist knowledge which has only been available to a few. Over the years, doctors have assumed a position of power and superiority towards their patients. Doctors operate within strict ethical guidelines but there is an assumption that only the doctor (or other healthcare professional) has the right information so they decide what their patient needs without necessarily having to discuss and agree it with them. Historically, it has been a one-sided relationship in which the doctor decided the when, what and how of the therapy. According to Funari (2005), the patient was not a subject of treatment but an object of that treatment.

Recent research and best practices highlight the need for practitioners to develop empathy and the psycho-social relationship with the patient. It is important that practitioners see their patients not as 'an intellectual curiosity' but as a *human being*. Each human being is unique; we have emotions, values, needs, preferences aligned to our family, social contexts and influences that differentiates each of us from every other.

The aim of this chapter is to highlight the need for attitudinal and cultural changes in doctors and other healthcare professionals, for example by improving practitioners' literacy in terms of their self-awareness and awareness of others. It offers some practical tools to improve skills regarding listening, empathy and the ability to ask questions. In doing this, the practitioner supports the patient to build a critical awareness of their reality, in which they have an opportunity to describe their emotions, values and needs. It provides time to recognise their resources and implement relevant actions that lead them to co-create the process of care, wellbeing and often healing.

Awareness of oneself and of others: emotional intelligence (EI) and empathy

Awareness is a broad concept that includes several aspects of the human essence including psychological (thoughts), behavioural, emotional and spiritual levels of our being. Important perspectives of this for medical and healthcare practitioners are those of emotional intelligence (EI) and empathy.

EI is a mix of several competences that are deeply intertwined and focused on our capacity of managing our own emotions and those of other people in a functional way.

Emotional intelligence consists of two main areas:

- Intrapersonal: the ability to acknowledge what happens inside ourselves (self-awareness) and to act functionally (self-management)

- Interpersonal: the ability to recognise others' emotions, what happens within relationships (others' awareness) and to act functionally with others (relationship management)

One particular aspect of EI that is crucial within a therapeutic partnership for generating patient empowerment is empathy. Empatheia derives from the ancient Greek inside and pathos meaning feeling or pain. Empathy is the ability to recognise emotions, attribute a mental state and respond appropriately. Empathy has several definitions and is often confused with taking other people's emotions/pain upon oneself. This interpretation is far from being correct. Empathy according to Baron-Cohen and Wheelwright (2004) is the *"drive or ability to attribute mental states to another person/ animal and entails an appropriate affective response"*. It is an ability to recognise the emotions of others.

Empathy is one of the emotional behaviours that we possess. The confusion with the interpretation of this word derives from its similarities with sympathy. Sympathy is created when the emotions and feelings of one person generate the same ones in another person, establishing a shared emotional status.

Empathy represents a concept of 'healthy emotional closeness'. In this way, the practitioner can 'recognise and embrace the patient's emotions' and, at the same time, be aware that they are not theirs. This is a different emotional status from that of being affectionate (sympathetic) or fond of someone. In this condition, should unpleasant emotions occur, we embrace the pain and we truly feel the other person's mood.

Empathy in the medical field can, therefore, clearly bring advantages with the creation of a relationship that seeks to understand, representing an act of empowerment itself. On the other hand, by basing the relationship on affection, doctors and healthcare practitioners take the patient's emotions on themselves risking a very likely burnout. Burnout is the lose-lose, with the practitioner not being useful to themselves or to the patients. Several studies have been conducted that demonstrate the benefits of an empathetic approach with the therapeutic relationship. These include a series of positive outcomes such as: better ability to follow the treatment, better therapeutic cohesion, more satisfied patients, fewer hospitalisations due to complications and less legal actions between patients and doctors.

The good news is that empathy is a skill that can be developed, perhaps finding ways to use our mirror neurones in a way that benefits practitioners and the patient. There is a need for practitioners to enhance self-awareness and take steps to allow growth both as a person as well as a professional.

Attending to these perspectives can have significant advantages in the doctor-patient relationship, especially if we take into consideration the uncertainty and impact of particular medical diagnoses and treatments. Emotions may be running high in our patients. The ability that we possess to manage our emotions and motivate ourselves constitutes the so-called interpersonal skills. Developing interpersonal skills, including empathy, enables practitioners to recognise and be with other people's emotions and respond appropriately.

Social skills are also important for communication. Generative communication, such as exploring thinking, attitudes and behaviours and managing conflict and uncertainty then create a collaborative discussion where the practitioner and patient work as a team. Self-awareness and ability to self-regulate are crucial elements to be able to adapt and create the empowering relationship. These are important aspects of emotional intelligence.

Listening: THE expertise

Listening is the most important part of the communication process. From the combined personal experiences as a doctor, coach and trainer, the following pillars of effective communication in medicine were identified as shown in the figure.

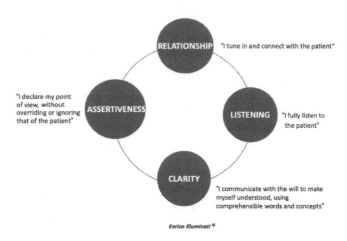

Figure 6: A model of communication skills in medicine

Following this model allows us to work together with the patient, and importantly not interrupt. Several studies have noted short interruption times. The first in 1984 (Howard Beckman and others) found an average of just 18 seconds before the doctor interrupted the patient while they were describing the reason for their appointment. In 1999, a repeat study demonstrated an interruption time of 21 seconds. Similar studies conducted in 2018 showed an average interruption rate of 11 seconds, with some discrepancies between family doctors and specialists. When doctors are asked what prevents them from fully listening to their patients, the usual and most common answer is, *"Time! I have very little time for my appointments and a lot of patients have to sit outside and wait!"*

If listening is crucial when a lot of time is available, it is vitally important when typically practitioners only have a few minutes.

Listening fully refers to the quality of the listening. Humans have five different listening levels that are ranked from the least to the most effective:

- Passive – we are busy or distracted and our attention is elsewhere

- Fake – not interested, pretending to listen

- Selective (usually the most common one) – we are thinking about what we would say/answer

- Active – we are truly listening to what they say and putting our thoughts aside

- Empathic listening – we feel/embrace the emotions

The danger we have as practitioners is to switch continuously from passive listening (looking at records/notes, filling in documents etc) to selective listening, which in the 'expert's' mindset often means 'I have enough information to evaluate possible problems and solutions as well as potential treatments'. The disadvantage of this behaviour is that the practitioner may lose important information that might be extremely useful to simplify the patient journey from the diagnosis to the treatment.

Listening fully means to listen actively and empathetically. Being alongside the patient, gathering and clarifying all the information. Once there is clarity, the practitioner can engage with their expert mindset and maintain their relationship with the patient.

Building communication skills in this way builds strong relationships and the capacity of the patient to follow through with medical recommendations and it:

- avoids misunderstandings and conflicts
- reduces the chance of errors based on practitioner assumptions
- establishes trust and shows that you care in a therapeutic partnership
- increases the likelihood of obtaining useful information
- allows co-creation of a viable treatment plan

Coaching questions: the art of creating patient empowerment

Using coaching skills is an essential process to support empowerment. It brings critical awareness, alignment on motivation between patient and practitioner and action (see Cycle of Empowerment, Chapter 1). Coaching as defined by the ICF (International Coach Federation) is *'partnering with individuals in a thought-provoking and creative process that inspires them to maximise their personal and professional potential'*.

Typically, a medical consultation will focus on clinical scenarios, possible diagnoses or more detailed examinations and treatment options. If our questions are mainly anamnestic, they may not take into account other aspects that are crucial for successful treatment. It is necessary to explore the patient's motivations, and delve deeper to discover what knowledge of the disease they have and establish their desired end goal. In addition, the practitioner needs to be confident that the patient has fully understood their recommendations by asking pertinent coaching questions.

An excellent example outlined by Schutz and colleagues of the coaching approach in the medical field can be found by the use of Motivational Interviewing as outlined as important patient-centred guidelines for managing obesity in primary care. This approach explores motivations and readiness to change.

There are three keys to potential success:

1. The perceived importance of change must be high.

2. The patient feels confident in his/her ability to change behaviour.

3. This change is a priority for the patient; it's the right moment to do it,

This is an example of using a coaching approach that has been widely adopted in the healthcare field. With the use of a total listening approach for communication and the coaching skill of creating the relationship, patients become empowered and more likely adhere to their therapy.

A consequence of this approach is that such a complete interview would require additional time and longer time slots for doctors' appointments. However, if doctors master the basic principles of coaching, they could insert in a very natural way some questions within the process of anamnestic questioning. The potential benefits of such an approach may include avoiding wasting time, granting a better patient journey and a more effective treatment.

Examples of questions extracted from Motivational Interviewing are:

- How are you feeling about X at this time?

- How important is it for you to change your behaviour now?

- What stressful events are there in your life at the moment that could be a barrier to change?

- If you decide to change your lifestyle, what would you change?

- What are some reasonable goals you could set regarding X?

- What kind of changes would you be willing to start with?

- What kind of help would you like to meet your goals?

Top Tips to improve your patient empowering skills

To wonder for yourself:

1. What is my goal and my purpose with the patient?

2. What is my belief about empathy?

3. When interacting with the patient, how much of the time am I listening to/empathically compared to other ineffective levels? How could I improve? (if necessary)

4. How could I integrate coaching questions into my clinical practice?

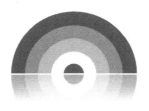

CHAPTER 10

COHERENCE: OPTIMAL HEALTH THROUGH BREATHWORK, EMOTION REGULATION AND BIOFEEDBACK

Gavin Andrews

"Feelings come and go like clouds in a windy sky. Conscious breathing is my anchor." Thich Nhat Hahn

Breathing – we all do it. Emotions and feelings – we all have them. From the first moments of our birth to the last seconds of our life we are breathing and feeling. We are experiencing emotions *in utero* well before our birth too.

How we breathe and the variety, frequency and intensity of the emotions we feel are foundational to our physical and mental health. While there might not be a perfect way to breathe, nor a perfect mix of emotions, there are definitely more and less optimal ways of breathing and feeling.

This chapter explores how we can empower our own and our patients' health by consciously regulating both breath and emotions to create an optimal, scientifically measurable state called psychophysiological coherence (coherence for short). As with the other approaches in this book, empowerment is the outcome of increased awareness, practical information and learning of new responses, in this case, coherence.

It is important to clarify that experiencing negative and unpleasant emotions is normal and that they serve important purposes. We are not advocating the regulation of all negative emotions. What we are advocating is self-awareness of emotions and self-regulation when they are not appropriate or helpful to the situation and when they are being experienced too frequently and intensely. Experiencing too much negative emotion is damaging to our physical and mental health and quality of life. Emotion regulation is a learnable skill and is essential to healthy adaptation, recovery from stress and longevity. Coherence is an important foundation for emotion regulation.

What is coherence and why is it important?

Coherence can have profound benefits for physical and mental health and quality of life.

Coherence has a variety of meanings. In common use it generally means clarity of thought and communication or unified wholeness. In physics, coherence refers to harmonious, ordered and energy-efficient synchronisation within a system or between systems. We can think of humans as a whole system made up of a number of integrated sub-systems such as cardiovascular, respiratory, nervous, digestive, endocrine etc. These sub-systems are regulated by homeostasis and coherence practice appears to restore and sustain homeostasis, thereby helping the body and brain to repair and revitalise itself. Sustained or frequent stress – physical, mental, emotional or existential – creates wear and tear (allostasis) which, over time, will result in physical and/or mental health problems. Coherence practice is therefore a way to consciously reduce stress and increase health and resilience.

How can we create coherence?

We can all intentionally create coherence and with practice we can increase our levels of coherence. Through this we can begin to create a new unconscious baseline of coherent physical and mental functioning. The good news is that it is really quite simple to do. Coherence can be initiated by regulating your breathing and increased by intentionally experiencing positive and pleasant emotions.

Breathing – the way into coherence

Firstly, you need to learn how to optimise your breathing. Research shows that breathing slowly and deeply at a rate of around six breaths per minute quickly shifts most people towards coherence. Six breaths per minute equates to a 10-second breath cycle. Most people breathe far too quickly and shallowly with the average person taking between 12 to 20 breaths per minute. Breathing at six breaths per minute is the most effective rate for creating coherence within the autonomic nervous system and between heart and brain, and inducing feelings of calm alertness.

You should breathe in and out through your nose, not your mouth. Nasal breathing kills more bugs, allows more oxygen into the blood and creates 50% more resistance than mouth breathing. This extra resistance gives your heart and lungs a workout and keeps them strong and healthy.

Deep, slow, nasal breathing at a cycle rate of around 10 seconds also has a profound impact on physiology. It quickly increases your Heart Rate Variability (HRV); this means that there are greater variations in the beat to beat changes in your heart rate. It also shifts your heart's rhythm into coherence. This means that your heart rate is progressively speeding up and slowing down in a repeating pattern. The heart produces the strongest electrical signal in the body and, when coherent, the heart rhythm oscillates at a frequency of 0.1 Hertz (Hz). Brainwaves synchronise to the 0.1 Hz oscillations and synchronisation spreads to other areas of the brain including the prefrontal cortex. As activity increases in your prefrontal cortex and decreases in your stress centres, it improves your capacity for self-awareness and self-regulation of feelings, thoughts and behaviours.

The figure below presents a simplified illustration of what happens when someone realises that they are stressed and then practises coherent breathing.

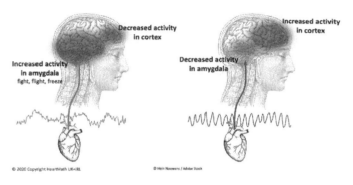

Figure 7: Coherent breathing and the stress response

During physical, mental and emotional stress our body and brain shifts into fight, flight, freeze mode and our heart's rhythms become more chaotic (incoherent). Our heart sends incoherent signals to the brain which sustains increased activity in our stress centres and reduces activity in our prefrontal cortex. Our skills of self-awareness and self-regulation are compromised when our prefrontal cortex is less active. Stress affects our brain a bit like a lobotomy, albeit a reversible one. However, if you are aware that you are stressed, coherent breathing can enable you to change the communication quickly between your heart and brain. Your coherent heart rhythms change the information going to your brain. The activity in your stress centres quickly reduces and as a result, increases in your prefrontal cortex. This then facilitates emotional and behavioural self-regulation.

Emotion regulation – taking coherence to the next level

Many forms of psychological therapy, such as Cognitive Behavioural Therapy (CBT), rely on using the prefrontal cortex to change thoughts and thereby change emotions and behaviours. Of course, this 'top down' approach can work, but during significant stress it can become very difficult because the activity in your prefrontal cortex is significantly reduced. In effect your stress centres are overpowering your prefrontal cortex. This is why stress often causes us to do or say things we later regret once stress has subsided.

Coherent breathing puts your prefrontal cortex back in control. This means you can now intentionally choose to experience a different emotion. Positive emotions increase coherence and prefrontal activity further than breathing alone.

Positive and pleasant emotions such as care, appreciation, gratitude and compassion are particularly helpful in social situations or relationships with others and they also have physiological benefits.

The figure below presents a simplified description of how coherence practice works as a 'bottom up' physiology-first approach. It can also complement and elevate the effectiveness of 'top down' cognitive therapies. An increasing number of therapists and health professionals are integrating coherence training into their approaches.

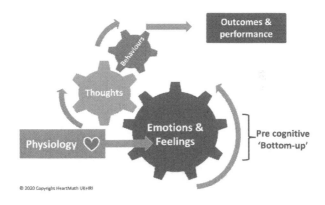

© 2020 Copyright HeartMath UK+IRI

Figure 8: The interplay between physiology and performance

Coherence techniques

The following three techniques were developed by HeartMath®, a company founded in 1991 and headquartered in California, USA. HeartMath conduct coherence and HRV (Heart Rate Variability) research and innovate HRV biofeedback technologies.

Heart-Focused Breathing™

This technique is the foundation for coherence building. It is a simple, eyes-open, in the moment technique and can be done at any time, especially when experiencing stress. This technique will quickly reduce the activity in your brain's stress centres. It will also significantly reduce the production of adrenaline and cortisol.

- Step 1: Focus your attention in the area of your heart or centre of your chest

- Step 2: Imagine that your breath is flowing into and out of your heart or chest area, breathing deeply but comfortably

Try breathing at a pace of five seconds for the in-breath and five seconds for the out-breath. If that feels uncomfortable then breathe a little faster or slower but try to keep your breath balanced, smooth and sustained. Placing your hand on your heart can help with maintaining your focus there. Ensure that your belly is relaxed so that your diaphragm can move fully.

This method of breathing can be done throughout the day and is appropriate for many if not most situations which require you to be calm and to perform cognitively.

Quick Coherence®

This technique builds upon Heart-Focused Breathing to include the shift into a positive or pleasant emotion. The positive emotion increases coherence further and can potentially add other physiological benefits.

These include the release of hormones including Dehydroepiandrosterone (DHEA), which is important for health and vitality, and oxytocin, which promotes pro-social behaviour and can buffer the stress response. Again, it is an eyes-open, in the moment technique and can be done at any time. It is particularly useful as a way to prepare for a challenging situation, to recover quickly after stress and as a way to top up resilience throughout the day. It begins with steps 1 and 2 above and then includes a third step:

- Step 3: Recall someone or something in your life for which you feel genuine care, appreciation or gratitude; breathe the feelings in and out

Heart Lock-in®

This technique is more like a traditional meditation in that it requires you to sit quietly in a comfortable place and to dedicate a good amount of time, eg 10-20 minutes or more. It is similar to the Buddhist meta or compassion meditation and is designed to help you practise feeling care and compassion for yourself and for others. Research also shows that this technique can significantly change HRV and hormonal baselines and also benefit anxiety, depression and Post Traumatic Stress Disorder (PTSD).

- Step 1: Focus your attention in the area of your heart or centre of your chest; imagine that your breath is flowing into and out of your heart or chest area, breathing deeply and comfortably

- Step 2: Activate and sustain a regenerative feeling such as love, appreciation, care or compassion
- Step 3: Radiate that renewing feeling to yourself and others

Using biofeedback to train coherence

Many people are not interested in, and may even be resistant to, the idea of breathwork, emotion regulation and meditation. Additionally, many people who do give them a go find it too difficult or struggle to notice benefits. This is often because they lack interoception (awareness of internal bodily states). They may give up too quickly instead of persevering to create a habit, develop their interoception and experience the cumulative benefits of consistent practice.

HRV Biofeedback can be a very effective way to get people interested in coherence practice and to help them develop awareness of physical, mental and emotional states, obtain information and validation while practising, and learn how to get better.

Summary

Breath and emotions are unconscious reactions. But they can also be conscious choices too. Practising coherence techniques, with or without biofeedback, provides a simple and effective way to shift the ratio of unconscious reactions towards more conscious choices.

We all have to breathe, and we can't avoid feeling. If we want to live a healthier and happier life, and we want the same for our patients, then we will all benefit from spending more of our time breathing and feeling coherently.

Top Tips

1. Become more conscious of your breathing.

2. Breathe through your nose, slowly and deeply and balance your in and out breaths.

3. Become more conscious of your emotions.

4. Exercise your choice to feel pleasant, positive emotions like care, appreciation, gratitude and joy.

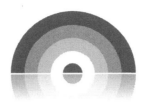

CHAPTER 11

MEASURES OF HEALTH

Ann Lewis and Christopher Ullman

"The groundwork of all happiness is good health." L Hunt

In our modern, busy and frequently pressured lives, we often pay little attention to our health and assume that as long as we do not have any symptoms of illness and we feel generally OK, then we are healthy. We visit our general practitioner (GP) only when we are presenting with symptoms and are looking for a diagnosis and medicine to alleviate the symptoms or to cure the illness.

On occasions we are offered health checks at our GP or through our workplace, which is good, as this encourages us to keep in mind the importance of staying healthy and, seeing data about ourselves with recommendations on how to optimise our health scores, can be motivating and empowering. Furthermore, in today's world, it is becoming very important to act before illness takes hold; remember the adage 'prevention is better than cure'.

With knowledge comes empowerment

Having an understanding of what measures to take, how they relate to your health and how changes to your diet and lifestyle will help to improve your health status gives you the ability to take control of your health. Then, by taking action and optimising your health, you will feel better, be more energised and importantly will become more resilient to communicable diseases such as viral infections. In addition, you will help to avoid non-communicable diseases such as type 2 diabetes mellitus, certain cancers, metabolic syndrome, Alzheimer's disease etc.

Inflammation

One of the key risk factors underlying these diseases is chronic low-grade inflammation. This can build up in the body over many years, but is symptomless, so you will be unaware of an issue. But over time this inflammation increases your risk of illness. Chronic low-grade inflammation can be assessed by measuring hsCRP (high sensitivity C-Reactive Protein) in a blood sample; however, this is not a common test and ideally it should be used in conjunction with other markers to assess inflammation.

However, a good surrogate marker is a simple measure of the amount of fat in your body (compared to your muscle mass). Inflammation affects the way that your body utilises energy by affecting the blood sugar level control and appetite control systems, making it hard to lose body fat. In fact, inflammation actually causes your body to lay down fat. This inflammation is often a result of a diet consisting of high levels of processed foods, but it can be addressed by changes in diet and reducing fat mass. Furthermore, stress has been shown to produce chronic low-grade inflammation, so it is important to look after all aspects of your life by actively participating in health empowerment.

The build-up of chronic low-grade inflammation in the body becomes a vicious cycle, causing fat deposition, which is itself inflammatory.

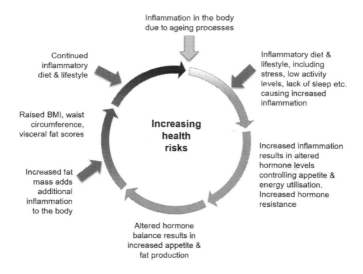

Figure 9: The vicious cycle of inflammation

Simple measures of health

There are many measures of health, some are easily collected yourself using apps and personal monitoring and tracking devices, but others will require turning to a healthcare provider. The first one that most people will likely know is the recommendation to do 10,000 steps/day. Although this figure has no real scientific basis, beyond comparisons with activity of hunter gatherers, the idea that people set themselves activity goals is good. The most important thing is to not be sedentary and to make sure that you move around and use your muscles as much as possible.

A recent study of older women found that those who managed 4,400 steps/day had lower mortality rates four years later than those averaging 2,700 steps/day, with the benefit plateauing at 7,500 steps/day. It is increasingly recognised that muscle strength enables individuals to maintain independence in later years. Building and maintaining muscle mass is also very important in reducing health risks.

We are also familiar with weighing ourselves, but the reason we do this is often not associated with being healthy, but because individuals want to improve their appearance, eg to drop a dress size. But your weight, or specifically the amount of body fat and muscle you have, are key markers of health. Too much body fat causes health risks, whereas a good proportion of muscle promotes good health. A familiar estimate of body fat is BMI (Body Mass Index) which is calculated from your weight and height. Many modern sets of scales will give you this reading when you weigh yourself and it is a good indicator of your overall health. For example, a BMI of 18.5 to 25 is considered healthy and levels above this range can highlight when the body is overly fat. But if you have a very muscular physique your BMI will be raised as well, so treat this data in the context of your physique.

The unhealthiest fat is visceral fat which is found around your middle and is laid down around your internal organs. Evidence suggests that having high amounts of visceral fat makes you more susceptible to type 2 diabetes mellitus (T2DM). Some modern scales or body composition analysers will give you a visceral fat score, but if you do not have access to these, a simple way of determining if visceral fat is an issue is to measure your waist and hip circumference. The healthy ratio for your waist-to-hip is ideally in the range 0.7 to 0.9 for men and 0.65 to 0.85 for women; higher than this indicates that you may have too much visceral fat and reducing this by dietary changes and exercise would be beneficial.

Cardiovascular risk

Simple measures of blood pressure are useful as they can highlight cardiovascular issues and, along with BMI, cholesterol ratio and lifestyle information can be used to assess heart age and cardiovascular risk. Lipid levels can be used to track health and frame cholesterol in a meaningful context. The best self-test lipid monitors give readings of HDL, commonly called good cholesterol, as higher levels are associated with a lower risk of heart disease, and LDL bad cholesterol, as high levels increase the risk of cardiovascular disease. It is the ratio of these two lipoproteins, which are the main components of total cholesterol, which give valuable information on health status and risk. The levels of these lipids in your blood can be optimised by good nutrition and exercise.

Diabetes risk

An easy way to assess your diabetes risk is to use the online Diabetes UK Risk Score (https:// riskscore.diabetes.org.uk). Diabetes occurs when your body can no longer control blood sugar levels with the hormone insulin. The onset of type 2 diabetes mellitus (T2DM) is promoted by long-term high production of insulin as a result of poor diet and over-consumption of highly refined carbohydrates (eg sugar) and exacerbated by chronic low-grade inflammation. This is usually avoidable with good diet and lifestyle, and hence can be reversed if the contributing factors are addressed early enough.

The Diabetes UK Risk Score uses measures of excess weight gain (waist measurement and BMI), family history, ethnicity and associated health problems such as high blood pressure and your risk can be tracked over time. In conjunction with this, a measure of your HbA1c level can be very useful as this will give information on your average blood sugar levels over the previous three months and can highlight if you have a healthy control of your blood sugar levels. If not, you may be pre-diabetic or have tipped over into diabetes, in which case you will need to speak with your GP. Another familiar test is the measure of fasting glucose and this provides a measure of your ability to control your blood sugar on that day. Both of these tests can be determined from a finger prick blood test.

Vitamin D

There are many tests available for key micronutrients (vitamins and minerals), and these tests would help you to understand any deficiencies in your diet. A key nutrient for health is vitamin D and a lack of this vitamin is associated with several disorders such as metabolic and cardiovascular diseases. This essential vitamin can be obtained from oily fish, egg yolks and fortified cereals, but is also made by the skin as a reaction to sunlight, so sensible exposure to the sun is good for health. In the winter taking a vitamin D supplement eg cod liver oil is often advised.

A healthy lifestyle and diet are key

It is never too late, or too early, to find out how healthy you are and how well you are ageing. Listen to your body; if you are tired, have poor sleep, feel hungry all the time, struggle with your weight, then your body is not functioning at its best. Take control of your health by measuring and tracking your health status with easy body measures. Invest in or try to find access to a body composition analyser which will give you fat and muscle mass measures and may also give you a visceral fat score, and measure these regularly.

Introduce as much activity into your lifestyle as you can. This will not only help your physical health but your metal wellbeing.

Eat well by planning your meals well ahead and keep your food cupboards stocked up with a range of quality, nutritious foods and snacks. Recommendations for five-a-day of vegetables and fruit is a simplification of the healthy eating index (HEI) which sets recommendations for food groups. Eating a balanced diet is recommended with less than 10% of energy being derived from added sugars. Taking advice from a nutritional therapist can be very helpful or, if you find behaviour change particularly difficult, then wellbeing coaches will be able to help you make positive changes.

Top Tips

1. Take time to think about your health and how well you are ageing – listen to what your body is telling you.

2. Make small improvements to your diet and lifestyle – these can have a big impact on your future health.

3. Take simple body measures regularly – this will help you to understand and take control of your health.

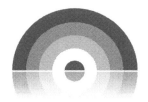

PART 3:
LEARNING

In the previous chapters you will have experienced a tour of discovery and learning. You will have gained an insight into the power of coaching interventions as a motivational and life-affirming methodology. Based on extensive research into the effectiveness of mindful awareness and present moment attention you have been introduced to new ways of being with your individuals/patients.

These empowering methods will contribute to the happiness, motivation and attitude for both yourself and your individuals/patients. Mind, body and spirit do not work in isolation, they are essential parts of the whole, combining to promote optimal health and wellbeing for all.

Learning is an ongoing process and needs commitment, reflection and regular practice.

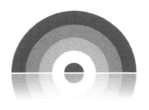

CHAPTER 12

COACHING SUPERVISION: MIND, BODY, METAPHOR

Jackie Arnold

This chapter explores the way in which coach supervisors create a safe space for supervision and nurture a genuine quality of present moment attention. Being present in the here and now combined with acceptance and non-judgment. By increasing your levels of attention, it becomes possible to co-create a deep-thinking space for the supervisee to reflect and grow.

It can also increase levels of attention and empathy for both supervisor and those seeking supervision.

You will discover Clean Language questions and Symbolic Modelling work of psychotherapist David Grove, and of Penny Tompkins and James Lawley who have been at the forefront of developing and promoting the application of Clean Language. A powerful intervention and valuable skill for coach supervisors, it enables you to stand back from your work with as little interference as possible. In this journey of discovery, we have a unique glimpse into the world of our supervisee, creating a strong bond and a true supervision partnership.

"The inner self is revealed in the unconscious language and symbolic landscape of the supervisor and their supervisee." Jackie Arnold, *Coaching Supervision at Its Best (2011)*

What you will discover in this chapter

- How to create a safe learning space and mindful presence – for both supervisor and supervisee

- How Clean Language and symbolic modelling can create different perspectives to facilitate learning in coaching supervision

Coach supervisors are trained to understand different energies in the environment and tap into another person's energy field. At the same time, they need to be acutely aware of diverse patterns of thought and their own energy flow. Only then can intrusions be put aside and the focus be entirely on the other person and their landscape, co-creating a transformative mindful space. Paying respectful attention to the body movements, the sighs, the breathing and the voice tone of the supervisee. This allows you to access your own intuition, self-manage and trust that what arises in the session is there for a reason. Expectation and preconceived ideas about how the session should go are left at the door.

It becomes apparent long after the sessions that this transformative relationship is carried further. Supervisees are better able to reflect on their own learning and discoveries and take away new understanding to their own coaching practice. Only when nurturing this special connection, keeping out your own ego and intrusive thoughts, can learning and supervision be truly effective.

When you tap into the silence that quietens you down, it enables you to go deeper into the soul of your sessions. It enhances the capability to 'hold' the different parts of the system and to be acutely aware of what is often *not* said. This calm space and sharp focus ensures contractual boundaries are not crossed and all stakeholders (relationships) are respected.

It is this quality of mindful attention that shows respect and allows for an unconditional positive space for supervisees to explore and grow. When you pay attention and are present in the 'now' of the session you can support supervisees to clarify their own understanding of those sometimes very complex contexts.

Sometimes we only see elements of these multiple facets and complexities and therefore as Peter Senge says:

"The key to 'seeing from the whole' is developing the capacity not only to suspend our assumptions but to 'redirect' our awareness towards the generative process that lies behind what we see."

Clean Language

Clean Language was devised by psychotherapist David Grove. It is a way to keep assumptions out of interactions with individuals so you can work directly with your perceptions. It consists of approximately 30 questions, asked in a curious way and with a particular tone of voice. The pace and timbre of the voice is a key element in the effectiveness of Clean Language questions. The slow pace and brevity of clean questions enables supervisees to delve safely into the situations they bring to sessions. It frees the chatter and allows for a mindful approach. This slowing down and coming into the present moment is enhanced by the pauses between our questions and the reflecting back of the supervisees' exact words.

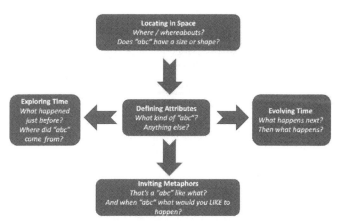

**Figure 10: The original nine-questions compass
(note: 'abc' are the individual's exact words)**

When using Clean Language in coaching supervision it is particularly useful to develop the metaphors that supervisees use naturally as they speak. The supervisor, by asking clean questions, helps to slow the supervisee down and gets them to think about what they really mean by the words they've used. Their metaphors are unique to each supervisee and as they are developed by the supervisor, the supervisee unconsciously feels understood. They feel their own view of the situation has been acknowledged.

Case study: Supervision – the place of 'not knowing'

This case study looks at one of a series of six coaching supervision sessions (session 3 of 6) that will illustrate the importance of bodily presence and 'staying with' the supervisee.

This coach was a highly experienced person working in the health sector wishing to develop her own coaching practice. She was also managing the transition to coach from a successful career as a senior grade nurse. She was motivated and wanted to use supervision to enhance her coaching style and build her practice. After the first two sessions where clear contracting had been agreed and the sessions planned with a suitable venue identified, a concern began to emerge in the mind of the developing coach.

At the beginning of the third session it was apparent that the coach had not been able to align her previous role with that of her new role as a coach. She was fearful (her words) of stepping out of her 'safe' environment into one that appeared totally new and unknown. It is often challenging to 'stay with' a supervisee in the space of not knowing. However, it is at these crucial junctions that mindfulness and presence, two of the essential management tools of a supervisor, are at their most powerful. Exploring the fear and staying out of the supervisee's way using Clean Language (see below) during this exploration proved to be a real turning point.

Using a basic Clean Language question (see diagram for clean questions) I asked *"if there was anything else about this fear she had identified and if it had a size or shape (prompting her to move to a symbolic or metaphorical description by describing it visually)."* There was a long silence and then she told me that *"the fear was a pink blob at the front of her forehead."*

Consciously re-grounding and by calm breathing to keep focused on her phrases, I asked her *"what kind of blob this was when it was 'pink and at the front of her forehead'."* She replied that it was like a piece of *'rubber'* that could be different shapes and she could move it where she wanted. I had no idea where she was in her thoughts or feelings, so stayed with her in her metaphorical landscape both with my energy and the slow pace of my voice. She said it felt as if this had given her back the power she had lost. The fear was no longer *'looking over her shoulder'* as before but out there in front where she could move it. To explore this metaphor further I asked *"when the pink blob was where she could move it, and it was no longer looking over her shoulder, and she had the power back… what happened then?"*

After a longish pause and a few further questions, she said her fear was no longer in control of her. She realised the only person who was able to hold her back was herself. She then spoke about her coaching practice with renewed enthusiasm and identified specific ways forward for the coming weeks.

In this session the coaching space of 'not knowing' created a catalyst for a real shift of energy for the supervisee. This was unfamiliar territory in that she was encouraged to visualise her fear as something tangible/visual and to explore it in a totally new way. She had no notion of where the pink rubbery fear had come from. She had merely discovered she had a choice: to allow it to stop her from moving forward or to put it where she could move and control it.

In this case study the power of investigating the metaphorical landscape of the supervisee allowed essential new knowledge to emerge.

Metaphors

Everyone uses metaphors as part of daily life regardless of their cultural background, they are familiar to us and form part of who we are.

"The essence of metaphor is understanding and experiencing one kind of thing in terms of another." George Lakoff & Mark Johnson

Examples in English are: I'm at a loss, light at the end of the tunnel, banging my head against a brick wall, ball-park figure, price fall/rise, it's a crying shame, I'm feeling down... etc.

One supervisee described his situation in a company as that of "a lion trainer trying to tame the lions"; when he noticed and investigated this further, he realised his vision of his individuals may not have been helpful or appropriate!

Benefits of using Clean Language

The benefits of using Clean Language in coaching supervision are that we enable supervisees to think and reflect on their behaviour and actions without language interference. We empower them to own the metaphors they come up with and take them away for further reflection. The ideas supervisees generate through the use of metaphor are generally quite inventive and idiosyncratic. They stay with the supervisee who generates them and provide an anchor a long time after the sessions. Supervisees get to understand the structure of their own thinking and behaviour patterns and how these impact on their individuals. It increases their self-awareness and provides the support for exploration into the complex areas of their work.

When stepping into the role of supervisor, letting go of your own fear of making the right intervention or asking the right question will greatly enhance the symbolic modelling process. When you are mindful of your own chatter and can relax and 'let go to let come' you become physically still and more attuned to the present moment. Using Clean Language and metaphor is powerful in allowing you to stand back, observe and respectfully challenge the supervisee when appropriate.

The questions and interventions all arise from the supervisee and their words. When this is done with courage and moment to moment awareness, there is a fluidity and simplicity in the way images occur. Your journey together co-creates this safe reflective space while discovering other landscapes and adding new learning and perspectives.

Top Tips

1. Getting fluent in Clean language and Symbolic Modelling takes time and patience; just use what you feel comfortable with and keep it simple.

2. When supervising at your best, create a deep heartfelt and respectful connection with supervisees by coming to sessions calm and prepared.

3. Mindfulness and deep breathing will bring your own emotions under control so creating a safe environment.

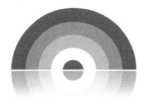

CHAPTER 13

COLLABORATIVE LEARNING AND DEVELOPMENT: THE PROCESS OF EMPOWERMENT

Andrew A Parsons, Jackie Arnold and Sue Jackson

"Learning can be defined as any process that in living organisms leads to a permanent capacity change and which is not solely due to biological maturation or ageing." Knud Illeris

Coaching conversations create a psychologically safe environment for the individual to explore and challenge perspectives. The practitioner has a role to co-create the reflective environment and facilitate learning and change. The changes sought by the individual may be goal based, for example they seek to change a behaviour or attain specific objectives. Individuals may be clearer on what they don't want. In our experience, coaching conversations often start by exploring these issues when individuals are faced with a challenging professional, personal or health situation and their future feels uncertain and filled with many unknowns.

This is especially the case working at the Fountain Centre. Individuals living with and beyond cancer often face a number of changes that results in them needing to transition from their familiar ways of living to something new. Our coaching conversations are therefore frequently focused on the individual learning how to acknowledge the reality of their situation and negotiate barriers to fully realise potential.

Both these goal- and development-based outcomes of coaching conversations feature within the Professional Charter for Coaching and Mentoring and in competency-based approaches to accreditation with several professional bodies.

Mentoring conversations may also use coaching approaches. However, mentoring differs from many coaching approaches in that it specifically offers the practitioners' experience. According to the Professional Coaching and Mentoring Charter (see references), it can be defined as:

'The transfer of knowledge or skill from a more experienced to a less experienced person through learning dialogue and role modelling.'

In the context of empowerment in health and wellbeing, the cycle of empowerment provides a framework for both the coaching and the mentoring process. In line with the three pillars of awareness, information and learning described in Chapter 1, coaching and mentoring approaches may support the individual developing competence and confidence in specific techniques. Typically, these approaches build and maintain your critical awareness, expand the range of your choices and your capacity to respond to change (a fundamental part of learning). For example, mindfulness and other grounding techniques may be very useful skills for your client to develop. Becoming proficient in these approaches enables them to expand their awareness and develop clarity on future intentions and goals. Additionally, conversations regarding nature, spirituality, nutrition and the ways our body work provide resources and fruitful opportunities for reflection, development and support in the management of their lives.

Supporting our individuals to learn also provides our own learning process in line with the three pillars. Reflection, continual professional development and supervision are an essential part of our development as practitioners, occurring in parallel to the development of those we work with.

Learning requires application

Adult Learning Theory has core dimensions that operate in a cyclical and dynamic process including the ways individuals acquire knowledge based on the stimulus for change (learning) and the interaction with their environment.

To illustrate this process, we can consider a common stimulus in our coaching at the Fountain Centre, where coaching provides individuals with emotional support.

The individual may be receiving or have completed life-changing medical treatment following a cancer diagnosis. In this situation there are many unknowns. Often the individual knows and expresses what they don't want. They may describe this as a desire to 'move on' following treatment. They can feel 'lost' and unsure of ways to bring this about, and this desire for change or to 'move on' creates a stimulus for learning that might trigger them seeking professional support. Exploring 'moving on' is a vital part of the coaching contract and for many people (in our experience) this means feeling like they are playing an active part in their lives again, that is, becoming empowered in their health, wellness and relationships.

Theoretically the acquisition of learning is dependent on content (eg knowledge, skills, attitudes) and the incentive to learn. Our incentives will dictate how much energy we will put into the uncomfortable (requiring energy) process of learning. The first role of the practitioner is to create the safe, confidential learning environment for the individual's exploration and development. Co-establishing the working relationship with transparent agreements and expectations of each other can change the dynamics and responsibilities of the coaching relationship for the individual and reduces the appearance of defence mechanisms or barriers to learning. Establishing this working relationship is essential to develop the learning programme.

The cycle of empowerment provides a framework for the practitioner and individual. The framework could feature as part of the agreement, a process by which the individual has some control over the conversations that will provide opportunities for the collaboration. The dialogue that is generated through coaching creates awareness of intentions, attitudes and behaviours. It develops learning and formulates the emerging plans and actions. In the coaching process we explore narratives and perspectives and support the emergence of the individual's goals. These coaching interventions also support the individual to develop their resources and promote their competence.

Learning outcomes

The different types of learning and the individual barriers to learning are important areas for the practitioner to be aware of and negotiate. Consideration also needs to be given to the social and diverse cultural aspects of learning.

Learning is a multi-dimensional life-long process. In our early years we learn things in isolation and gradually bring them together to create our picture of the world. This type of learning also occurs in adults (eg learning a

PIN number) and is seldom the main topic of our work in supporting people develop empowerment. They are not so interested in mechanically learning isolated information that may not be utilised in their lives.

The more common form of assimilative learning allows people to add new information to existing schemas to improve efficiencies and activities and may not relate to different contexts. In this regard, individuals may develop skill in a range of immediate self-help techniques such as meditation or breath techniques. These self-help techniques allow people to better manage and regulate their thoughts, feelings and emotions. Individuals find that developing awareness and proficiency in self-management techniques often helps them focus. This area of skill development may even feature as part of the professional contract and provide alignment on immediate/interim goals and motivations.

The more demanding transcendent learning takes place when existing schemas or models are challenged by the coaching or mentoring sessions and new ones created. This process takes more energy as it is re-creating a different perspective and thinking about the world. These types of learning may also be understood as single- and double-loop learning. Double-loop learning takes place when the learner thinks about and challenges their own views and beliefs. When this type of learning occurs at the level of personal identity values, a transformational learning can take place. This type of learning is less frequent than the others and occurs when a major challenge to the person's self-concept is generated. These often occur around a significant life event, for example retirement, redundancy, divorce or a life-changing medical diagnosis such as cancer. The transition that results may need considerable amounts of energy to negotiate, which can be shared and supported significantly in a coaching environment. Transparency and clarity of these types of learning outcomes are an essential part of the relationship.

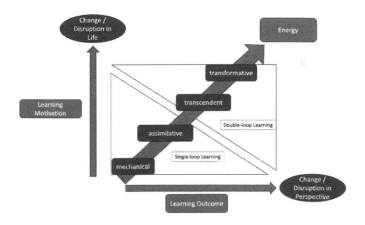

Figure 11: Schematic representation of the interplay between motivation for learning, outcomes and type of learning experienced (adapted from Illeris, 2018a)

Negotiating barriers to learning across different situations and environments

To create change the learner needs to overcome learning barriers including the defence mechanisms they have in place. As we develop, we build a range of assumptions that we use to negotiate our lives. When we come across new information that does not quite fit to the expected assumptions, humans tend to reject or modify the information so it fits with their current view of the world. One of our roles as practitioners is to reflect to our individuals their existing words, behaviours and actions to increase their awareness of resources and barriers and explore different perspectives and possibilities. Our beliefs in their ability to do so will also likely pay dividends for the individual.

As coaches or mentors we work also with the resistance of learners (individuals) to change. Building new perspectives often brings 'active' resistance from the learner as they attempt to hold on to the status quo. The skilled practitioner can support the individual to recognise this and can negotiate and expand possibilities with different coaching approaches. This refers to the individual style of practitioner and also the abilities of the learner, and how these fundamental changes in perspective may operate in the different parts of their lives. Systems approaches for understanding feedback loops and various coaching tools such as the Wheel of Life and Neil's Wheel (see Resources) offer the opportunity for all individuals regardless of culture, education or background to safely explore different perspectives.

It is also worth noting that within the coaching and mentoring relationship that is built on trust and openness there is a two-way process of learning. The individual's learning is focused on ways they can change their perspectives to reach their new emergent goals and through this process to move towards their potential. For the practitioner, despite being on the same path of empowerment in health and wellness, professional learning comes through the creation of an environment that enables the individual to overcome passive and active barriers to learning. Joint learning occurs when they partner to facilitate the individual's ability to embed that learning in the different contexts of their lives.

Bringing empowerment to life through coaching

The three core coaching pillars of awareness, information and learning provide an empowering, collaborative and parallel process for the practitioner and individual.

For the individual

The process enables the individual to develop a critical awareness of their situation and develop powerful motivation to consciously select, implement and review their choices. Developing the ability to self-regulate and self-manage through and from this process empowers the individual in their life and situation.

For the practitioner

The coaching process entails the practice for the coach of developing and honing awareness of personal state and the ability to stay in the moment with their individual. This gives rise to heightened presence. Awareness in coaching improves trust, non-judgment, curiosity and attention. It creates an environment in which what is happening for the individual, for self and in the dialogue is explored and acknowledged (internally and/or through the process). The skills to hold these simultaneous processes brings insight, flexibility and adaptability to the coaching. It helps practitioners to challenge our assumptions. It promotes empathetic and compassionate support for the individual and for self as practitioner.

The parallel process

The parallel learning processes of individual and practitioner occurs through engaging with the empowerment cycle. Contained within the perspective of parallel process is the idea of the transference and counter-transference phenomena. Here we hold the possibility that each participant in the coaching relationship will react and respond in ways that are outside conscious awareness. For example, in any learning situation there are possibilities for shame, guilt and fear to be evoked. Some of these less easy feelings to acknowledge may emerge and belong to earlier learning situations.

As both parties become more aware, trusting and at ease with sharing what arises in the coaching relationship, the work will flow out of the current reality and not out of the past. Both the individual and the practitioner are likely to be dealing with a range of human emotions including shame, guilt and fear. As outlined above, the parallel process of learning and empowerment is occurring in both parties. For the practitioner, they have the additional dimension of holding the coaching and mentoring process whilst also developing through supervision, albeit at a later date.

The coaching/mentoring dialogue expands and deepens learning through sharing, offering, self-managing and enquiring together to serve the needs of the individual, the coach and the process.

Managing boundaries of practice

A critical competency in supporting individuals at the Fountain Centre is to be aware of our boundaries of practice. It is an essential part of both coaching and mentoring professional practice and work within the NHS.

Within the Centre we are fortunate to come under clinical governance which enables us to work effectively with other services in the Centre and the wider hospital. Healthcare professionals signpost or refer to the coaching service and we have ready access to guide our individuals to other services. The definition of the boundaries of our practice is a key learning area for the practitioners. An analysis of our experience showed that volunteer coaches had experience of working with people with health conditions and were trained in self-help stress management techniques. In our co-supervision (reflection and learning) group, we often explore these professional and therapeutic boundaries.

The Health Awareness Tool (see Corrie, 2019, Corrie & Parsons [in press]) is an approach to guide coaches in working with mental health and is a useful tool to support these discussions. The model is not a diagnostic tool, however it provides a framework to consider the types of conversations we are having with our individuals. It encourages the practitioner to be aware of what is and is not said. Bringing awareness to the levels of functioning and resources discussed in the conversation helps practitioners develop four main types of interaction. Those where the individual develops four groups of conversations through Flourishing (High Functioning & Resources), Managing (High Functioning & Low Resources), Existing (Low Functioning & High Resources) and Struggling (Low Functioning & Resources).

Typically, coaching and mentoring conversations are thought to occur with individuals who are flourishing and here coaching can continue. A heightened awareness of the role of coaching needs to be questioned by both practitioner and individual in dialogue for the Managing and Existing groups. Active monitoring of the practice in these groups benefits both individual and practitioner in the collaborative learning endeavour. For example, if the individual is Struggling in terms of their functioning and their resources, it is highly appropriate to question the learning approach offered by coaching. Learning requires agency and energy and these may be in short supply for them. As practitioners, the management of our boundaries of practice develops with every professional and supervisory experience.

Supporting individuals to make significant adjustments and changes to their lives (eg following redundancy, divorce, other medical diagnoses or career changes) can be thought of as therapeutic work. It is therefore important to ensure that we, as practitioners, are looking after ourselves, managing our stressors and what arises in coaching with suitable recovery and attention to our physical, mental, emotional and spiritual lives. The awareness and self-compassion generated through mindfulness practice and the Attitudinal Foundations of Mindfulness can be of particular support for this.

Boundary management and awareness of personal processes are also important for healthcare practitioners and organisational leaders and managers in their coaching and mentoring roles. This is important for our professional standards, our awareness of workplace stress, mental health triggers and to comply with legislation.

Conclusions

Heightened listening skills enable the practitioner to focus on the narratives of the individual, the current story of their life and how this might be recognised, learned from and released to generate a new narrative which has a more empowering purpose.

This process engages values, assumptions, beliefs and self-leadership strategies to provide opportunities for transcendent and transformative learning in the enabled learner. The integration of learning is a collaborative endeavour. The key learning dimension of integration requires action, communication and cooperation which are all leadership skills that can be developed. Indeed, supporting our individuals to negotiate their barriers to a learning environment is often an important part of the coaching contract. Transformation of personal narratives requires integration within the social and professional systems of the individual.

Using Freire's definition of empowerment has enabled us as practitioners to develop a cycle of empowerment pertinent to coaching. The key phases align well with professional coaching/mentoring competencies, they provide a framework for learning, personal leadership and the development of coaching skills to support salutogenic (health promoting) action.

Top Tips

1. Keep reflecting on your practice.

2. Use supervision regularly.

3. Focus on continual improvements.

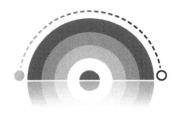

CHAPTER 14

ENDINGS AND NEW BEGINNINGS

Jackie Arnold, Sue Jackson and Andrew A Parsons

We hope you will have gained insights from our shared knowledge, enthusiasm and experience. We are all dedicated to developing working relationships with clients which fit their needs, hopes, challenges and lives to empower and enable their self-management. In doing so we hope they will have the opportunity to enhance their independence and the relationships in their lives. In a world facing significant challenges, such as viral pandemics, climate change and global uncertainties, individuals, communities and workplaces need resources to feel empowered and not depleted.

Empowerment supports:

- individual and community health and wellness

- effective management of the demands within health provision services including the emerging models of Lifestyle Medicine and Social Prescribing

- the attainment of the UN Sustainable Global Goal 3: Good Health and Wellbeing

Our book illustrates how our different experiences of coaching and mentoring enables empowerment and results in improved self-management and personal development.

This increases society's capacity for health and wellness.

Our objectives in creating this publication were to share skills and learning, improve community health and wellbeing in alignment with the UN and heightens our own skills for positive impact for our cancer patients and their families at the Fountain Centre.

We hope the book provides insights and learning for fellow professionals who support the health and wellness of others and advances some self-help techniques for everyone to use.

While the passion to write this book came from our skills in coaching in cancer, we firmly believe these approaches are transferable. Developing the skills to manage challenging transitions and develop or grow from the experience is relevant to many life-changing experiences, health conditions and all walks of personal and professional life.

If you would like to engage and expand your competence and confidence to work in this area, please contact the relevant author or the editors.

REFERENCES

Change and Complexity: The challenges to 'health' in the 21st century

Barber, H.F. (1992). Developing strategic leadership: The US army war experience. *Journal of Management Development, 11*, 4-12.

Bauer, G., Davies, John K. & Pelikan, J. (2006). The EUHPID Health Development Model for the classification of public health indicators. *Health promotion international, 21*(2), 153-159.

Brown, V.A., Harris, J.A. & Russell, J.Y. (2010). *Tackling wicked problems through trans-disciplinary imagination.* London: Earthscan.

National Wellness Institute: https://nationalwellness.org/

World Health Organization. (2004, 20 December 2019). Promoting mental health: Concepts, emerging evidence, practice: Summary report. Retrieved from https://www.who.int/mental_health/evidence/en/promoting_mhh.pdf

World Health Organization. (2014, 20 December 2019). Basic documents. Retrieved from http://apps.who.int/gb/bd/PDF/bd48/basic-documents-48th-edition-en.pdf#page=1

Empowerment Defined

Anderson, R.M. & Funnell, M.M. (2010). Patient empowerment: myths and misconceptions. *Patient education and counselling, 79*(3), 277-282.

EPF. (2017). Toolkit for Patient Organizations on Patient Empowerment. Retrieved from https://www.eu-patient.eu/globalassets/library/publications/patient-empowerment-toolkit.pdf

Freire, P. (1970). *Pedagogy of the oppressed.* New York: Continuum.

Freire, P. (2019). *Pedagogy of the Heart.* London UK: Bloomsbury Academic.

Spreitzer, G.M. (2008). Taking stock: A review of more than twenty years of research on empowerment at work. In J. Barling & C.L. Cooper (Eds.), *Handbook of organizational behavior* (Vol. 1, pp. 54-72). Thousand Oaks CA USA: Sage.

Spreitzer, G.M. (1995). Psychological empowerment in the workplace: Dimensions, measurement and validation. *Academy of Management Journal, 38*(5), 1442-1465.

Coaching Enables Learning and Empowerment

Cox, E., Bachkirova, T. & Clutterbuck, D.A. (2014). *The complete handbook of coaching.* London: Sage.

David, S., Clutterbuck, D. & Megginson, D. (Eds.). (2016). *Beyond goals: Effective strategies for coaching and mentoring*. Abingdon UK: Gower.

Palmer, S. & Whybrow, A. (2018). *Handbook of coaching psychology: A guide for practitioners*. Abingdon UK: Routledge.

Sforzo, G.A., Kaye, M.P., Todorova, I., Harenberg, S., Costello, K., Cobus-Kuo, L. & Moore, M. (2018). Compendium of the health and wellness coaching literature. *American journal of lifestyle medicine, 12*(6), 436-447.

Spence, G.B. & Deci, E.L. (2016). Self-determination theory within coaching contexts: Supporting motives and goals that promote optimal functioning and wellbeing. In S. David, D. Clutterbuck & D. Megginson (Eds.), *Beyond goals: Effective strategies for coaching and mentoring* (pp. 85-108). Abingdon UK: Gower.

Wolever, R.Q., Simmons, L.A., Sforzo, G.A., Dill, D., Kaye, M., Bechard, E.M. & Yang, N. (2013). A systematic review of the literature on health and wellness coaching: defining a key behavioural intervention in healthcare. *Global advances in health and medicine, 2*(4), 38-57.

Awareness

Presence and mindfulness

Arch, J.J. & Craske, M.G. (2006). Mechanisms of mindfulness: Emotion regulation following a focused breathing induction. *Behaviour research and therapy, 44*(12), 1849-1858.

Dane, E. & Brummel, B. J. (2014). Examining workplace mindfulness and its relations to job performance and turnover intention. *Human Relations, 67*(1), 105-128.

Hall, L. (2013). *Mindful coaching: How mindfulness can transform coaching practice.* Kogan Page Publishers.

Halpern, B.L. & Lubar, K. (2004). *Leadership presence.* Penguin.

Harland, P. (2012). *TRUST ME, I'M THE PATIENT Clean Language, Metaphor and the New Psychology of Change.* London England: Wayfinder Press.

Janki, D. (2011). *365 Days of wisdom: Daily messages to inspire you through the year.*

UK: O Books.

Janki, D., Vegso, P. & Johnson, K. (2015). *Feeling great: Creating a life of optimism, enthusiasm and contentment.* Deerfiled Beach, FL USA: Health Communications Inc.

Nhat-Hanh, T. (1995). *The miracle of mindfulness: An introduction to the practice of meditation.* Beacon Press.

Nhat-Hanh, T. (2010). *Peace is every step: The path of mindfulness in everyday life.* Random House.

Tolle, E. (2004). *The Power of Now: A guide to spiritual enlightenment.* New World Library.

Grounding yourself in times of chaos

Clond, M. (2016). Emotional freedom techniques for anxiety: a systematic review with meta-analysis. *The Journal of nervous and mental disease, 204*(5), 388-395.

Feinstein, D. (2019). Energy psychology: Efficacy, speed, mechanisms. *Explore, 15*(5), 340-351.

Maharaj, M.E. (2016). Differential gene expression after Emotional Freedom Techniques (EFT) treatment: A novel pilot protocol for salivary mRNA assessment. *Energy Psychol Theory Res Treat, 8*(1), 17-32.

Stapleton, P. (2019). *The science behind tapping: A proven stress management technique for the mind and body.* Carlsbad, CA USA: Hay House, Inc.

Possibilities of using our bodies to empower us

Levine, P.A. (2010). In an unspoken voice: How the body releases trauma and restores goodness. Berkley, CA USA: North Atlantic Books.

Van der Kolk, B. (2014). The body keeps the score: Mind, brain and body in the transformation of trauma. USA: Penguin.

Nature and spirituality

Conway, P. & Hefferon, K. (2019). The extraordinary in the ordinary: Skychology - an interpretative phenomenological analysis of looking up at the sky. Retrieved from https://www.researchgate.net/publication/331702864_The_extraordinary_in_the_ordinary_Skychology_-_an_interpretative_phenomenological_analysis_of_looking_up_at_the_sky

Global Wellness Summit. (2020). Retrieved from https://www.globalwellnesssummit.com/wp-content/uploads/2020/01/GlobalWellnessTrends2020.pdf

Jackson, S. (2005). The Potential on the Doorstep: The Importance of Gardens in the Psychological Wellbeing of Older People. *J. Ther. Hort*, 16, 28-37.

Kabat-Zinn, J. Retrieved from https://www.habitsforwellbeing.com/nine-mindfulness-tips-from-jon-kabat-zinn/

Kabat-Zinn, J. (1996). *Full catastrophe living: How to cope with stress, pain and illness using mindfulness meditation.* London UK: Piatkus.

Kaplan, S. (1995). The restorative benefits of nature: Toward an integrative framework.

J. Environ. Psychology, 15, 169-182.

Spencer, M. (2012). What is spirituality? A personal exploration. Retrieved from https://www.habitsforwellbeing.com/nine-mindfulness-tips-from-jon-kabat-zinn/

Stevenson, M.P., Schilhab, T. & Bentsen, P. (2018) Attention Restoration Theory II: a systematic review to clarify attention processes affected by exposure to natural environments. *J. Tox. and Environ Health*, 21, 227-268.

Ulrich, R.S. (1984). View through a window may influence recovery from surgery. *Science, 224*(4647), 420-421.

Perspectives on building a healthy immune system

Childs, C.E., Calder, P.C. & Miles, E.A. (2019). Diet and immune function. *Nutrients,* 11. Doi: 10.3390/nu11081933.

Hato, T. & Dagher, P.C. (2015). How the innate immune system senses trouble and causes trouble. *Clinical Journal of the American Society of Nephrology,* 10, 1459-1469.

Mantis, N.J., Rol, N. & Corthésy, B. (2011). Secretory IgA's complex roles in immunity and mucosal homeostasis in the gut. *Mucosal immunology,* 4, 603-611.

Marcos, A., Nova, E. & Montero, A. (2003). Changes in the immune system are conditioned by nutrition. *European journal of clinical nutrition,* 57, S66-S69.

Minihane, A.M., Vinoy, S., Russell, W.R., Baka, A., Roche, H.M., Tuohy, K.M., Teeling, J.L., Blaak, E.E., Fenech, M. & Vauzour, D. (2015). Low-grade inflammation, diet composition and health: current research evidence and its translation. *British Journal of Nutrition,* 114, 999-1012.

Nicholson, L.B. (2016). The immune system. *Essays in biochemistry,* 60, 275-301.

Popkin, B.M., D'anci, K.E. & Rosenberg, I.H. (2010). Water, hydration and health. *Nutrition reviews,* 68, 439-458.

Information

Coaching for Personal Leadership – an essential approach to health in times of change and uncertainty

Antonovsky, A. (1979). *Health, stress and coping.* San Francisco: Jossey-Bass.

Antonovsky, A. (1987a). Health promoting factors at work: the sense of coherence. In R. Kalimo, M. El-Batawi & C.L. Cooper (Eds.), *Psychosocial factors at work and their relation to health* (pp. 153-167): World Health Organization Geneva, Switzerland.

Antonovsky, A. (1987b). *Unraveling the mystery of health: How people manage stress and stay well.* San Francisco: Jossey-Bass.

Antonovsky, A. (1996). The salutogenic model as a theory to guide health promotion. *Health promotion international, 11*(1), 11-18.

Bauer, G., Davies, J.K. & Pelikan, J. (2006). The EUHPID Health Development Model for the classification of public health indicators. *Health promotion international, 21*(2), 153-159.

Behrendt, P., Matz, S. & Göritz, A.S. (2017). An integrative model of leadership behavior. *The leadership quarterly, 28*(1), 229-244.

Bridges, W. (2003). *Managing transitions: making the most of change* (2 ed.). New York, NY: Da Capo Lifelong Books.

Corrie, S. & Parsons, A.A. (in press). Emerging conversations about the role of coaching in mental health. In M. Watts & I. Florance (Eds.), *Emerging conversations in coaching*. Hove, East Sussex: Routledge.

Deci, E.L. & Ryan, R.M. (1985). *Intrinsic motivation and self-determination in human behavior*. New York: Plenum.

Deci, E.L. & Ryan, R.M. (2008). Self-determination theory: a macrotheory of human motivation, development and health. *Canadian Psychology, 49*. doi:10.1037/a0012801.

Dodge, R., Daly, A., Huyton, J. & Sanders, L. (2012). The challenge of defining wellbeing. International Journal of Wellbeing, 2(3), 222-235.

Dolbier, C.L., Soderstrom, M. & Steinhardt, M.A. (2001). The relationships between self-leadership and enhanced psychological, health and work outcomes. *The Journal of Psychology, 135*(5), 469-485.

Drath, W.H., McCauley, C.D., Palus, C.J., Van Velsor, E., O'Connor, P.M.G. & McGuire, J.B. (2008). Direction, alignment, commitment: Toward a more integrative ontology of leadership. *The leadership quarterly, 19*(6), 635-653.

Eriksson, M. (2017). *The sense of coherence in the salutogenic model of health.* In Maurice B. Mittelmark, Monica Eriksson, Jurgen M. Pelikan, Geir A. Espnes, Shifra Sagy, Georg F. Bauer & Bengt Lindstrom (Eds.), *The handbook of salutogenesis* (pp. 91-96). doi:978-3-319-04600-6_11.

Eriksson, M. & Lindström, B. (2005). Validity of Antonovsky's sense of coherence scale: a systematic review. *Journal of Epidemiology & Community Health, 59*(6), 460-466.

Eriksson, M. & Lindström, B. (2006). Antonovsky's sense of coherence scale and the relation with health: a systematic review. *Journal of Epidemiology & Community Health, 60*(5), 376-381.

Eriksson, M. & Lindström, B. (2007). Antonovsky's sense of coherence scale and its relation with quality of life: a systematic review. *Journal of Epidemiology and Community Health, 61*(11), 938-944. doi:10.1136/jech.2006.056028.

Illeris, K. (2018). *Contemporary theories of learning: learning theorists... in their own words.* Routledge.

Kabat-Zinn, J. (1990). *Full catastrophe living: using the wisdom of your body and mind to face stress, pain and illness.* New York NY USA: Delacorte Press.

Konradt, U., Brombacher, S., Garbers, Y. & Otte, K-P. (2019). Enhancing Student's Self-Leadership Through a Positive Psychology Intervention? A Randomized Controlled Trial Using an Idiographic Perspective. *International Journal of Applied Positive Psychology, 4*(3), 149-167.

Lindström, B. & Eriksson, M. (2005). Salutogenesis. *Journal of Epidemiology & Community Health, 59*(6), 440-442.

Manz, C.C. (1991). Leading employees to be self-managing and beyond: Toward the establishment of self-leadership in organizations. *Journal of management systems, 3*(3), 15-24.

Manz, C.C. (1986). Self-leadership: Toward an expanded theory of self-influence processes in organizations. *Academy of Management Review, 11*(3), 585-600.

Maykrantz, S.A. & Houghton, J.D. (2020). Self-leadership and stress among college students: Examining the moderating role of coping skills. *Journal of American College Health, 68*(1), 89-96.

Mittelmark, M.B. & Bauer, G.F. (2017). *The meanings of salutogenesis*. In Maurice B. Mittelmark, Monica Eriksson, Jurgen M. Pelikan, Geir A. Espnes, Shifra

Sagy, Georg F. Bauer & Bengt Lindstrom (Eds.), *The handbook of salutogenesis* (pp. 7-13). doi: 978-3-319-04600-6_2.

Neck, C.P. & Houghton, J.D. (2006). Two decades of self-leadership theory and research. *Journal of Managerial Psychology,* 21(4), 270-296.

Parsons, A.A. & Mariposa, B. (2016). *Leading with Presence: What it is, why it matters and how to get it.* St Albans UK: The Endless Bookcase.

Prussia, G.E., Anderson, J.S. & Manz, C.C. (1998). Self-leadership and performance outcomes: the mediating influence of self-efficacy. *Journal of Organizational Behavior: The International Journal of Industrial, Occupational and Organizational Psychology and Behavior, 19*(5), 523-538.

Ryan, R.M. & Deci, E.L. (2019). Brick by brick: The origins, development and future of self-determination theory. In *Advances in motivation science* (Vol. 6, pp. 111-156): Elsevier.

Shapiro, S.L., Carlson, L.E., Astin, J.A. & Freedman, B. (2006). Mechanisms of mindfulness. *Journal of clinical psychology, 62*(3), 373-386. doi:10.1002/jclp.20237.

Spence, G.B., & Deci, E.L. (2016). Self-determination theory within coaching contexts: Supporting motives and goals that promote optimal functioning and wellbeing. In Susan David, David Clutterbuck & David Megginson (Eds.), *Beyond goals: Effective strategies for coaching and mentoring* (pp. 85-108). Abingdon UK: Gower.

Spence, G.B. & Oades, L.G. (2011). Coaching with self-determination theory in mind: Using theory to advance evidence-based coaching practice. *International Journal of Evidence Based Coaching and Mentoring, 9*(2), 37–55.

Spreitzer, G.M. (2008). Taking stock: A review of more than twenty years of research on empowerment at work. In J. Barling & C.L. Cooper (Eds.), *Handbook of organizational behavior* (Vol. 1, pp. 54-72). Thousand Oaks CA USA: Sage.

Spreitzer, G.M. (1995). Psychological empowerment in the workplace: Dimensions, measurement and validation. *Academy of Management Journal, 38*(5), 1442-1465.

Stelter, R. (2014). Third generation coaching: Reconstructing dialogues through collaborative practice and a focus on values. *International Coaching Psychology Review, 9*(1), 51-66.

Stelter, R. (2018). *The Art of Dialogue in Coaching: Towards Transformative Exchange.* Routledge.

Stelter, R. & Andersen, V. (2018). Coaching for health and lifestyle change: Theory and guidelines for interacting and reflecting with women about their challenges and aspirations. *International Coaching Psychology Review, 13*(1), 61-71.

Yukl, G. (2012). Effective leadership behaviour: What we know and what questions need more attention. *Academy of Management Perspectives, 26*(4), 66-85.

Patient-Centred Care: enhancing empowerment through shared decision making

Britnell, M. (2015). Transforming healthcare takes continuity and consistency. *Harvard Business Review, 28.*

Dilts, R. & Mazza, E. (2019). Success factors in healthcare. Retrieved from https://www.nlptrainings.gr/applications/success-factor-modeling-healthcare/

Elwyn, G., Durand, M., Song, J.J., Aarts, J.P., Barr, P., Berger, Z. & van der Weijden, T. (2017). A three-talk model for shared decision making: Multistage consultation process. *British Medical Journal, 359*, 1-7.

Elwyn, G., Frosch, D., Thomson, R., Joseph-Williams, N., Lloyd, A., Kinnersley, P. & Rollnick, S. (2012). Shared decision making: a model for clinical practice. *Journal of general internal medicine, 27*(10), 1361-1367.

Epstein, R.M., Mauksch, L., Carroll, J. & Jaen, C.R. (2008). Have you really addressed your patient's concerns? *Family practice management, 15*(3), 35.

IAPO. (2005). Declaration on Patient-centred healthcare: Patient-centred healthcare is the way to a fair and cost-effective healthcare system. Retrieved from https://www.iapo.org.uk/patient-centred-healthcare

Reid, P.R., Compton, D., Grossman, J.H. & Fanjiang, G. (Eds.). (2005). *Building a better delivery system: A new engineering/healthcare partnership.* Washington DC USA: National Academies Press.

Sharmer, O. (2018). *The essentials of theory U.* Oakland CA USA: Berrett-Koehler.

Stiggelbout, A.M., Van der Weijden, T., De Wit, M.P.T., Frosch, D., Légaré, F., Montori, V.M., & Elwyn, G. (2012). Shared decision making: really putting patients at the centre of healthcare. *BMJ, 344*, e256.

Triberti, S., Durosini, I. & Pravettoni, G. (2020). A 'Third Wheel' Effect in Health Decision Making Involving Artificial Entities: A Psychological Perspective. *Frontiers in Public Health, 8.*

Valentine, M., Nembhard, I.M. & Edmondson, A.C. (2015). Measuring teamwork in healthcare settings: a review of survey instruments. *Medical care, 53*(4), e16-e30.

Weller, J., Boyd, M. & Cumin, D. (2014). Teams, tribes and patient safety: overcoming barriers to effective teamwork in healthcare. *Postgraduate medical journal, 90*(1061), 149-154.

WHO. (2010). *Framework for action on interprofessional education and collaborative practice.* Geneva: World Health Organization Retrieved from https://bit.ly/3qnUyIM

Willard-Grace, R., Hessler, D., Rogers, E., Dubé, K., Bodenheimer, T. & Grumbach, K. (2014). Team structure and culture are associated with lower burnout in primary care. *The Journal of the American Board of Family Medicine, 27*(2), 229-238.

The Doctor's Role in Patient Empowerment

Baron-Cohen, S. & Wheelwright, S. (2004). The empathy quotient: an investigation of adults with Asperger's syndrome or high functioning autism, and normal sex differences. *Journal of autism and developmental disorders, 34*(2), 163-175.

Del Canale, S., Louis, D.Z., Maio, V., Wang, X., Rossi, G., Hojat, M. & Gonnella, J.S. (2012). The relationship between physician empathy and disease complications: an empirical study of primary care physicians and their diabetic patients in Parma, Italy. *Academic Medicine, 87*(9), 1243-1249.

Dornan, T. & Bundy, C. (2004). What can experience add to early medical education? Consensus survey. *BMJ, 329*(7470), 834.

Furnari, M.G. (2005). *Il paziente il medico e l'arte della cura.* Rubbettino Editore.

Goleman, D. (1996). Emotional intelligence. Why it can matter more than IQ. *Learning, 24*(6), 49-50.

Hojat, M., Louis, D.Z., Markham, F.W., Wender, R., Rabinowitz, C. & Gonnella, J.S. (2011). Physicians' empathy and clinical outcomes for diabetic patients. *Academic Medicine, 86*(3), 359-364.

Kendall-Raynor, P. (2007). Cautious welcome for plans to reform professional regulation. *Nursing Standard, 21*(25), 5-6.

Kennedy, C.M. (2004). A typology of knowledge for district nursing assessment practice. *Journal of Advanced Nursing, 45*(4), 401-409.

Maddocks, J. (2009). Creating an emotionally intelligent organisation. *The Coaching Psychologist, 5*(1), 27-32.

Maddocks, J. & Sparrow, T. (1998). The individual effectiveness manual. *JCA (Occupational Psychologist) Ltd.* Cheltenham, UK.

Paoli, L., Illuminati, E. & Falleri, A. (2011). *Il coaching per te*: Vallardi.

Rizzolatti, G. (2005). The mirror neuron system and its function in humans. *Anatomy and embryology, 210*(5-6), 419-421.

Schutz, D.D., Busetto, L., Dicker, D., Farpour-Lambert, N., Pryke, R., Toplak, H. & Schutz, Y. (2019). European practical and patient-centred guidelines for adult obesity management in primary care. *Obesity facts, 12*(1), 40-66.

Whitmore, J. (2002). *Coaching for performance*. UK: Nicholas Brealey Publishing London.

Wilson, J.H. & Hobbs, H. (1995). Therapeutic partnership: A model for clinical practice. *Journal of psychosocial nursing and mental health services, 33*(2), 27-30.

Coherence: optimal health through breathwork, emotion regulation and biofeedback

Bates, M.E., Lesnewich, L.M., Helton, S.G., Gohel, S. & Buckman, J.F. (2019). Resonance paced breathing alters neural response to visual cues: Proof-of-concept for a neuroscience informed adjunct to addiction treatments. *Frontiers in psychiatry, 10*, 624.

Fredrickson, B.L. (2012). *Positivity*. Oxford UK: One World.

Herrero, J.L., Khuvis, S., Yeagle, E., Cerf, M. & Mehta, A.D. (2018). Breathing above the brain stem: volitional control and attentional modulation in humans. *Journal of neurophysiology, 119*(1), 145-159.

Hinterberger, T., Walter, N., Doliwa, C. & Loew, T. (2019). The brain's resonance with breathing – decelerated breathing synchronizes heart rate and slow cortical potentials. *Journal of breath research, 13*(4), 046003.

Jentsch, V.L. & Wolf, O.T. (2020). The impact of emotion regulation on cardiovascular, neuroendocrine and psychological stress responses. *Biological Psychology*, 107893.

Kim, D., Kang, S.W., Lee, K-M., Kim, J. & Whang, M-C. (2013). Dynamic correlations between heart and brain rhythm during Autogenic meditation. *Frontiers in human neuroscience*, 7, 414.

Lehrer, P., Kaur, K., Sharma, A., Shah, K., Huseby, R., Bhavsar, J. & Zhang, Y. (2020). Heart Rate Variability Biofeedback Improves Emotional and Physical Health and Performance: A Systematic Review and Meta-Analysis. *Applied psychophysiology and biofeedback*. doi: 10.1007/s10484-020-09466-z.

McCraty, R. (2016). *Science of the heart volume 2*. Boulder Creek USA: Heartmath.

McCraty, R. & Shaffer, F. (2015). Heart rate variability: New perspectives on physiological mechanisms, assessment of self-regulatory capacity, and health risk. *Global advances in health and medicine*, 4, 46-61.

McCraty, R. & Zayas, M.A. (2014). Cardiac coherence, self-regulation, autonomic stability and psychosocial wellbeing. *Frontiers in Psychology*, 5, 1090.

Nhat-Hahn, T. & Laity, A. (1997). *Stepping into Freedom: Rules for monastic practice for novices*. Berkeley USA: Paralax Press.

Noble, D.J. & Hochman, S. (2019). Hypothesis: pulmonary afferent activity patterns during slow, deep breathing contribute to the neural induction of physiological relaxation. *Frontiers in physiology*, 10, 1176.

Schwerdtfeger, A.R., Schwarz, G., Pfurtscheller, K., Thayer, J.F., Jarczok, M.N. & Pfurtscheller, G. (2020). Heart rate variability (HRV): From brain death to resonance breathing at 6 breaths per minute. *Clinical Neurophysiology, 131*(3), 676-693.

Shahane, A.D., LeRoy, A.S., Denny, B.T. & Fagundes, C.P. (2020). Connecting cognition, cardiology and chromosomes: Cognitive reappraisal impacts the relationship between heart rate variability and telomere length in CD8+ CD28−cells. *Psychoneuroendocrinology, 112*, 104517.

Szulczewski, M.T. (2019). Training of paced breathing at 0.1 Hz improves CO2 homeostasis and relaxation during a paced breathing task. *PLoS ONE, 14*(6), e0218550.

Williams, C. (2020, 11 January). Easy ways to better you. *New Scientist,* 1.

Measures of Health

Guyenet, S.J. (2017). *The hungry brain: Outsmarting the instincts that make us overeat.* London, UK: Vermillion.

Harcombe, Z. (Ed.) (2017). *Diabetes unpacked.* Cwmbran: Columbus Publishing.

Spector, T. (2015). *The diet myth: The real science behind what you eat.* London, UK: Orion.

Learning

Coaching Supervision with Clean Language

Arnold, J. (2016). *Coaching skills for leaders in the workplace.* London UK: Robinson.

Arnold, J. (2014). *Coaching supervision at its BEST*: Crown House Publishing.

Bachkirova, T., Jackson, P. & Clutterbuck, D. (2011). *Coaching And Mentoring Supervision: Theory And Practice: The complete guide to best practice*: McGraw-Hill Education (UK).

Brown, K.W. & Ryan, R.M. (2003). The benefits of being present: mindfulness and its role in psychological wellbeing. *Journal of Personality and Social Psychology, 84*(4), 822-884.

Carroll, M. & Gilbert, M.C. (2005). *On being a supervisee.* London UK: Vukani.

Glickstein, L. (1998). *Be Heard Now: Tap Into Your Inner Speaker and Communicate with Ease.* Broadway Books.

Harland, P. (2012). *TRUST ME, I'M THE PATIENT Clean Language, Metaphor and the New Psychology of Change.* London England: Wayfinder Press.

Lawley, J. & Tompkins, P. (2003). *Metaphors in Mind: Transformation through symbolic modelling.* London UK: The Developing Company.

Murdoch, E. & Arnold, J. (Eds.). (2013). *Full Spectrum Supervision: Who you are is how you supervise.* St Albans UK: Panoma Press.

Orriss, M. (2006). Understanding the energetic principles that allow you to quantum coach. Retrieved from https://bit.ly/39UgMMr

Passmore, J. (2011). *Supervision in coaching: Supervision, ethics and continuous professional development.* Kogan Page Publishers.

Senge, P., Scharmer, C.O., Jaworski, J. & Flowers, B.S. (2004). Presence, Cambridge MA. *Society of Organizational Learning.*

Sullivan, W. & Rees, J. (2008). *Clean Language: Revealing metaphors and opening minds.* Camarthen, Wales: Crown House Publishing.

Collaborative Learning and Development: The process of empowerment

Argyris, C. & Schon, D.A. (1974). *Theory in practice: Increasing professional effectiveness.* Jossey-Bass.

Argyris, C. & Schon, D.A. (1978). *Organisational Learning.* Reading, MA: Addison-Wesley.

Capra, F. & Luisi, P.L. (2014). *The systems view of life: A unifying vision.* Cambridge University Press.

Clutterbuck, D. (2016). Working with emergent goals: A pragmatic approach. In *Beyond goals: Effective strategies for coaching and mentoring* (pp. 311-325). Oxford, UK: Gower.

Corrie, S. (Producer). (2019). What do Coaches Need to Know about Mental Health? *Webinar for the Special Group in Coaching Psychology*.

Corrie, S. & Parsons, A.A. (in press). Emerging conversations about the role of coaching in mental health. In M. Watts & I. Florance (Eds.), *Emerging conversations in coaching*. Hove, East Sussex: Routledge.

EESC. (2011). The professional charter for coaching and mentoring. Retrieved from: https://www.eesc.europa.eu/resources/docs/142-private-act--2.pdf

Hawkins, P. & Shohet, R. (2012). *Supervision in the helping professions*. Maidenhead, UK: McGraw-Hill Education (UK).

Illeris, K. (2018a). A comprehensive understanding of human learning. In K. Illeris (Ed.), *Contemporary theories of learning: Learning theorists... in their own words* (2nd ed.).

Illeris, K. (Ed.) (2018b). *Contemporary theories of learning: learning theorists... in their own words* (2nd ed.). London & New York: Routledge.

Karoly, P. (1993). Mechanisms of self-regulation: A systems view. *Annual review of psychology, 44*(1), 23-52.

Kegan, R., Congleton, C. & David, S.A. (2016). The goals behind the goals: Pursuing adult development in the coaching enterprise. In S. David, D. Clutterbuck & D. Megginson (Eds.), *Beyond goals: Effective strategies for coaching and mentoring* (pp. 229-244). Oxford, UK: Gower.

Kitchenham, A. (2008). The evolution of John Mezirow's transformative learning theory. *Journal of transformative education, 6*(2), 104-123.

Mezirow, J. (1991). *Transformative dimensions in adult learning*. San Francisco, USA: Jossey-Bass.

Mezirow, J. (2000). *Learning as transformation: critical perspectives on a theory in progress*. San Francisco, USA: Jossey-Bass.

Passmore, J. (Ed.) (2011). *Supervision in coaching: Supervision, ethics and continuous professional development*. London, UK: Kogan Page Publishers.

Spence, G.B. & Deci, E.L. (2013). Self-determination theory within coaching contexts: Supporting motives and goals that promote optimal functioning and wellbeing. In S. David, D. Clutterbuck & D. Megginson (Eds.), *Beyond goals: Effective strategies for coaching and mentoring* (pp. 85-108). Abingdon, UK: Gower.

Health and Wellness Resources

The Fountain Centre: https://www.fountaincentre.org

World Health Organization: https://www.who.int

Carers UK: https://www.carersuk.org/

Macmillan: https://www.macmillan.org

Marie Curie: https://www.mariecurie.org.uk/

National Hospice and Palliative Care:
https://www.nhpco.org

Working With Cancer:
https://www.workingwithcancer.co.uk

Kings Fund: https://www.kingsfund.org.uk

New Economics Foundation (2008). FIVE WAYS TO WELLBEING: Communicating the evidence
https://neweconomics.org/2008/10/five-ways-to-wellbeing-the-evidence

Mental Capital and Wellbeing Project (2008). Mental Capital and Wellbeing: Making the most of ourselves in the 21st century.
https://assets.publishing.service.gov.uk/government/uploads/system/uploads/attachment_data/file/292450/mental-capital-wellbeing-report.pdf

TOOLS AND OTHER RESOURCES

Examples of Professional Coaching Organisations

Association for Coaching:
https://www.associationforcoaching.com

European Mentoring and Coaching Council:
https://www.emccglobal.org

Health & Wellbeing Board Coaches:
https://www.nbhwc.org

International Coach Federation:
https://www.coachfederation.org

Medical Coaching Institute:
https://www.landing.mci-il.com

British Psychological Society Special Group in Coaching Psychology: htps://www.bps.org.uk

General Resources

Coaching at Work: https://www.coaching-at-work.com

VUCA – https://www.vuca-world.org

Variety of coaching skills and tools
https://www.businessballs.com

UN Sustainable Global Goals
ttps:// www.globalgoals.org

Self-Determination Theory
https:// www.selfdeterminationtheory.org

Patient Centred Care
https:// www.oneviewhealthcare.com

Emotional Intelligence see
https:// www.danielgoleman.info

The presence pyramid: See
https://theendlessbookcase.com/e-books/leading-
with-presence/

Coaching Tool: https://www.neilswheel.org

5 Ways to Wellbeing Planning Tool

Questions for your wellness strategy	5 ways to wellbeing developed by the New Economics Foundation See: https://neweconomics.org/2011/07/five-ways-well-new-applications-new-ways-thinking				
	Learn	**Connect**	**Be active**	**Notice mindfully**	**Give**
What is important about this for me?					
What will I do?					
When will I do it?					
Who will help me do it?					
If something gets in the way, how will I still do it?					
How will I know I am enjoying doing it?					
How will I learn to do it better next time?					

ABOUT THE AUTHORS

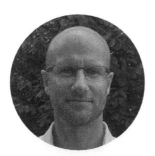

Gavin Andrews MBA, PGCHE

Gavin Andrews is the Managing Director of HeartMath UK and Ireland. His is also the founder of WeAddHeart, a global heart-focused meditation movement and a director of The Syntropy Partnership, a business which creates audio visual meditation aids.

In his role with HeartMath, Gavin trains coaches to use the HeartMath system within their practice and delivers training into organisations.

He lives in Surrey with his wife and children.

Email: gandrews@heartmath.co.uk

Instagram: heartmathuk

www.heartmath.co.uk

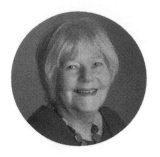

Jackie Arnold – ICF Accredited Coach and CSA Dip Coach Supervisor

Jackie runs her own coaching practice and holds a Certificate in Cancer Survivorship for Primary Care Practitioners. She founded the LinkedIn Cancer Coaching Community after her daughter's second diagnosis of cancer.

In addition to coaching in organisations, Jackie coaches cancer patients and their carers including volunteering at the Fountain Centre. She also holds regular Collaborative Coach Supervision Sessions.

Certified in Cognitive Behavioural Therapy, Transactional Analysis and NLP, Jackie integrates the powerful imagery and metaphors of Clean Language Methodology developed by David Grove. She believes this goes to the heart of issues, avoids assumptions, ensures respect and builds lasting trust and rapport.

She is the author of:

Coaching Skills for Leaders in the Workplace, Robinson 2016

Coaching Supervision at Its Best, Crown House 2015

Co-editor of CSA's *Full Spectrum Supervision*, Panoma Press 2016

Email: jackie@coach4executives.com

www.coach4executives.com

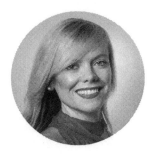

Victoria Hamilton – Registered Nutritional Therapist and Coach

Victoria's private practice, The Autoimmunity Nutritionist Clinic, specialises in autoimmune conditions and immune system health. Victoria is an advocate of the autoimmune protocol diet and is a certified AIP coach with a BSc Honours Degree in Immunology.

Victoria uses only scientific evidence-based nutritional therapies and protocols to help support these chronic conditions.

Victoria is passionate about health and wellness and has been able to manage the symptoms of her autoimmune conditions through adapting an AIP-inspired diet and engaging in lifestyle practices such as Pilates, meditation and walks in nature.

Email: victoria@theautoimmunitynutritionist.com

Instagram: @theautoimmunitynutritionist.com

www.theautoimmunitynutritionist.com

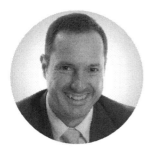

Enrico Illuminati MD – Executive Coach

Enrico is a GP with a medical degree. He was co-founder of a company in the field of Health and Fitness Medicine and Medical Director of a Clinical Centre in Milan.

He is currently Founder Partner of Sylenyx which provides coaching and training services in the Healthcare and Pharma environment.

An ICF Accredited Executive Coach (PCC) and expert in Emotional Intelligence, he is Certified for the Assessment 'Emotional Intelligence Profile' by JCA Occupational Psychologists (UK).

He has been a member of the faculty and trainer of numerous CME courses on issues concerning doctor-patient communication/relationship and the effectiveness of multidisciplinary teams. Enrico has been President Elect 2013 and President 2014 of the International Coach Federation – Italy.

He is co-author of the book *Il Coaching per Te* (Coaching for You) published in Italy.

www.sylenyx.com

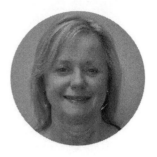

Sue Jackson BSc, MLD – AC Accredited Master Executive Coach and Accredited Coach Training Organisation

Sue is the Principal of Whitespace Coaching. She is an integrative coach, mentor, facilitator and trainer. Sue trains individuals, organisations and communities to develop coaching skills, which empower and enable adaptation, self-management and thriving. She creates a learning environment and a thinking space, based on trust, challenge and compassion.

Sue is the co-creator of the certified (AC) Salutogenic (Health and Wellbeing) Coaching programme.

Sue has expertise in mindfulness, mental health, cancer, vocational rehabilitation, emerging leadership and transition management. She is a volunteer virtual Fountain Centre coach and has a Certificate in Cancer Survivorship for Primary Care Practitioners.

Previous careers in and passion for biological science, horticulture, landscape architecture and education feed into her love of nature and its value for wellness, collaborations in research and her commitment to support individual and societal wellbeing.

Email: sue@whitespacecoaching.com

Instagram: @suejacksoncoach

www.whitespacecoaching.com

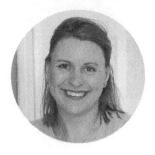

Aga Kehinde - Clinical Nurse Specialist and Performance Coach

Aga has 20 years' experience as a clinical nurse specialist in oncology and oncology research, she holds a diploma from The Coaching Academy in Personal Performance Coaching and Neuro-Linguistic Programming. Aga supports individuals who have experienced serious life challenges to navigate through the chaos, developing wellbeing strategies to reclaim purpose and meaning in their lives.

She is a cancer educator and a health and wellbeing lead for the Oncology Division at the Royal Surrey Hospital. She volunteers as a cancer coach at the Fountain Centre.

Aga created a hybrid approach that uses a full body-mind-energy experience for achieving holistic wellbeing. This combination of a lifetime experiences as a nurse with multiple techniques like Emotional Freedom Technique (EFT), Matrix Reprinting Technique (MRT) and NLP allows her to create an empowering model for self-development that her individuals desire.

Email: agakehinde@gmail.com

Instagram: @agakehinde

www.aga.kehinde.com

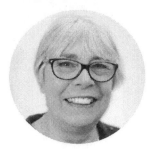

Ann Lewis - Managing Director and Scientist

Ann is a scientist with a special interest in healthy ageing and disease prevention. She has had a long career in the pharmaceutical industry, researching drug therapies across a range of medical conditions. Five years ago, Ann co-founded and became Managing Director for XenoVida Ltd, a healthcare company which delivers health status profiling and change support to individuals and to corporates who wish to support the health of their staff.

Ann has a keen scientific interest in promoting an understanding of the markers of health and in reducing health risks through simple dietary and lifestyle changes.

Email: info@xenovida.com

Instagram: xenovida.health

www.xenovida.com

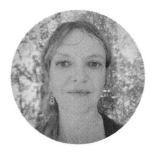

Silvia Mirandola – Biologist and ICF Accredited Coach

Silvia is a biologist with a PhD in Biomedical Sciences. She is an ICF Accredited Coach (ACC).

She has devoted 12 years to medical research and is author of several scientific publications.

She collaborated with different universities in Italy, London and New York. Later she moved to the pharma industry where she covered senior roles for nine years in the medical affairs of important multinationals.

In the last two years, Silvia has moved her interest in transformative leadership and team coaching programmes, designing and creating science-driven training and coaching services for sustaining high-performing teams in the healthcare system.

She is the creator of WeBiomimic© for Team Effectiveness, a team coaching game for managers based on the intelligence of nature and its strategies.

Email: s.mirandola@live.com

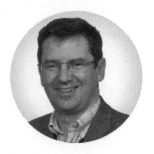

Andrew A Parsons MSc, PhD

Andrew works as a coach, trainer and mentor. He holds postgraduate degrees in Physiological Sciences (MSc, PhD) and Psychology (MSc). His practice supports people to adapt and thrive following professional and personal change. He is a volunteer coach at the Fountain Centre and experienced trainer.

He is certified in medical coaching, NLP, hypnotherapy, meridian therapies and HRV biofeedback. He is an EMCC Accredited Coach/Mentor at the Master Practitioner level. He takes an integrative and systemic approach that develops understanding of the self and relationship with teams, organisations, society and the environment.

He is the co-author of *Leading with Presence: What it is, why it matters and how to get it.* He has authored over 90 peer reviewed publications and contributed to educational literature in medicine, physiology and psychology.

Email: andrew.parsons@reciprocalminds.ltd

Instagram: reciprocalminds

www.reciprocalminds.com

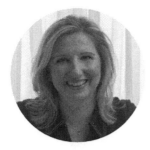

Fiona Stimson – Certified International Personal Performance Coach, Master of Neuro-Linguistic Programming and Master of Clinical Hypnotherapy

Fiona is 'The Kind Mind' Coach, supporting her individuals to live resourcefully, with purpose, compassion and authenticity, to achieve meaningful, lasting change personally and professionally for optimal health and wellbeing.

Inspired by her Mum's cancer journey and her own experiences on the importance of the mind and body interplay, Fiona coaches NHS professionals, senior leaders/managers and individuals impacted by cancer and chronic illness. Fiona has over 30 years' experience working in forensic science and healthcare as a scientist and senior leader.

Fiona is a coach and leader at The Royal Marsden Cancer Centre, she works as a volunteer coach at the Fountain Centre and runs her own private coaching practice at The Surrey Psychology Practice in Banstead, Surrey. Fiona is a finalist for the 2021 International

NLP Awards in the Healthcare category.

Email: hello@fionastimson.co.uk

Instagram: fionastimson

www.fionastimson.co.uk

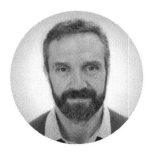

Chris Ullman PhD

Chris is Commercial Director at XenoVida Ltd, a company focused on improving health and wellbeing through the use of validated science. He has a BSc in Microbiology (University of Surrey) and a PhD in Biochemistry (University College London) from studying proteins of the immune system and cancerous proteins of papillomaviruses. He has over 20 years' experience of technology development and discovery in the biotechnology industry, specialising in biological therapeutics to fight cancer and other serious diseases. He has always maintained a keen interest in how to prevent, as well as cure disease, and the effects that diet and exercise have on our body. As an endurance 'athlete', he has recognised the importance of mental wellbeing and strength that is critical to support our physical health.

Email: info@xenovida.com

Instagram: xenovida.health

www.xenovida.com

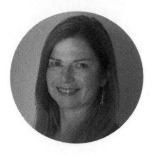

Amanda White - ICF and MCI Accredited Ontological Coach

As Director of Confluence Coaching Ltd, Amanda's mission is to support, motivate and inspire people whose journey through life involves change – adapting and thriving in new jobs, new cultures/countries, developing their leadership style, managing new life stages or challenges to their health and wellbeing.

Amanda is an experienced coach, accredited by the International Coaching Federation and the Medical Coaching Institute, with a background in corporate international human resources, mainly based in the pharmaceutical/healthcare industry. Through coaching and mentoring, Amanda encourages individuals to reframe challenges, seeing them from different perspectives and facilitating balance between logical thought, emotional input and physical impact. Individuals are supported to achieve well-considered balanced solutions while taking care of their personal wellbeing and resilience. Amanda coaches at the Fountain Centre.

Email: amanda@confluence-coaching.com

www.confluence-coaching.com